THE
OVERFAT
PANDEMIC

Exposing the Problem and Its Simple Solution
for Everyone Who Needs to

ELIMINATE EXCESS BODY FAT

DR. PHILIP MAFFETONE
Foreword by Lindsay Shaw Taylor

Skyhorse Publishing

> Disclaimer: This book should only be used
> as a reference and only used in the context of
> standard medical care with your physician.

Visit our website at www.skyhorsepublishing.com.

10 9 8 7 6 5 4 3 2

Library of Congress Cataloging-in-Publication Data is available on file.

Cover design by Tom Lau
Cover photo credit iStock

Print ISBN: 978-1-5107-2954-4
Ebook ISBN: 978-1-5107-2955-1

Printed in the United States of America

To all those committed to escaping the overfat pandemic.

And to the junk food industry—please help us release the world from the entangled trap of sugar addiction.

CONTENTS

CONTENTS

FOREWORD

As a psychologist turned health and fitness writer, I care deeply about helping people find a path to physical and mental wellness that is rooted in good science. Dr. Maffetone has been a trailblazer in the health and fitness world for decades. He has strongly influenced me professionally in my work with Primal Blueprint and personally with how my family and I eat and exercise. This book is his latest contribution to his revolutionary approach.

On the face of it, one might reasonably ask why we need another book on the topics of weight and weight loss (or fat and fat loss), diet, and exercise. The answer is because it is clear that many people still do not understand how to eat and move in ways that actually promote health, or they do not feel empowered to do so. As Dr. Maffetone correctly points out, the current system is flawed at every level, from industries that profit from people staying fat, to weight-loss approaches that we know don't work, to medical and governmental organizations promoting unhealthy food choices, to conflicting information about how to eat and exercise, to societal pressure to behave in ways that compromise health.

As a society, we are nowhere near a solution. In fact, as Dr. Maffetone argues, the problem hasn't even been properly *defined*; we are trying to fix the problem of *weight* instead of the problem of *fat*. Psychologists have long understood that what we call something matters. Language directs attention. When researchers are tasked with addressing weight problems, they will design interventions designed to move the number on the scale. Doctors become concerned, first and foremost, with how much their patients weigh. Individuals focus on this one single metric above all else. We all unintentionally lose sight of the real problem, so our remedies miss the mark.

Changing the focus from weight to fat is important, but of course it is not a panacea. Health professionals are still faced with the task of reversing the current pandemic not just by preventing more people from becoming overfat, but also by helping those who are already overfat change course. It is a task the community as a whole is clearly not equipped to handle at the moment. Unsurprisingly then, a lot of the blame is shifted to overfat individuals: Why don't people just eat better and exercise more? Don't they want to be thin and healthy?

Clearly those are the wrong questions to be asking. The overfat pandemic rages on not because of lack of motivation or lack of trying on the part of overfat individuals. Abundant evidence shows that most people want to be healthy, as well as to conform to societal standards of "acceptable," attractive bodies. Overfat individuals encounter tremendous stigma, from workplace and education discrimination, to prejudice in everyday social interactions. In a survey of over four thousand individuals, more than a third of those who were overweight (ranging from overweight to very obese) reported that they would sacrifice one year of life to not be obese; one in ten would sacrifice ten years.[1] (It is worth noting that *33 percent* of underweight respondents and 18 percent of normal-weight respondents would sacrifice ten years of life in order to avoid being obese.)

We know that most people who are overfat have tried many, many times to diet through calorie restriction, eating low-fat, low-calorie processed foods, and through extreme measures such as weight-loss pills, starving themselves, and purging. We also know this doesn't work. Their failure to lose weight is seen as *personal* failure, instead of a failure on the part of institutions and medical professionals to provide the right guidance. That is why books like this are so important.

The diet, fitness, medical, and pharmaceutical industries want people to believe that health is hard so we need their expert help, which undermines people's sense of agency with regard to their own well-being. The path forward involves empowering individuals to take control of their own health. This *must* include continuing to highlight the very real barriers to enacting these changes, including the addictive nature of sugar and grains, and the reality that the ability to make healthy food and lifestyle choices is constrained by economic inequality. It is important to keep reiterating that the industrialized food industry does not have our best interests at heart; it benefits from keeping us hooked and hungry, not nourished and satiated.

It also means challenging the tremendous dogmas around whole grains, fear of dietary fat, and a no-pain, no-gain mentality. The amount of bad information out there is disheartening to say the least, and much of it comes from people in positions of authority—doctors, government officials, and fitness professionals. By necessity, Dr. Maffetone and others in this sphere ask folks to reject conventional wisdom and do the opposite of what they have always heard is best for them. As we know well at Primal Blueprint, that can be a big hurdle. Going against the norm means making oneself *different*, which can be deeply uncomfortable, as well as logistically challenging in many ways. In the case of lower-carbohydrate, higher-fat eating, it means doing things that we have been told are *bad* for our health, like eating saturated fats. It also means *not* doing things we have been told are good for us, like eating "heart-healthy" whole grains and engaging in hardcore, sustained cardio workouts. This can provoke anxiety, fear, and uncertainty.

The way to overcome this so we as consumers feel emboldened to take our health into our own hands, and especially to reject what the masses are doing in favor of something that could actually work, is through education. It sounds trite, but knowledge is power; when the experts fail us, it is up to us to learn as much as we can and find a better way. We have control over many of the variables that affect our overall well-being, but messages like the one Dr. Maffetone offers—choose nourishing foods instead of junk, figure out what works best for you, and exercise in a way that fosters health instead of undermining it—can be drowned out by the noise of the same-old-same-old bad advice. Unless people who believe in his message keep repeating it over and over, loudly and with conviction, we will lose the message altogether.

Those of us with an interest in educating people about healthy lifestyles need to be intentional about how we talk to our audience, helping people understand not just what they need to do but *why*. We need to help grow communities of people dedicated to this way of eating and exercising so that individuals have social support, and their health-promoting choices are reinforced. Progress will require us to be diligent, but patient. The method that Dr. Maffetone prescribes in *The Overfat Pandemic* is simple, but the problem is incredibly complex. At every level, from governmental to corporate to community to family to individual, there are challenges. But as long as people like Dr. Maffetone continue to fight the good fight, offering a better way forward, I am hopeful for a healthier future.

—Lindsay Shaw Taylor, PhD (Social/Personality Psychology)
Senior Writer and Researcher, Primal Blueprint
Ultrarunner and Iron(wo)man

INTRODUCTION

TEN TENANTS OF OVERFAT

First, a personal story, which begins at birth, with a bottle of sugar water. It had a sexy name, even scientific-sounding: a glucose solution. This was my first food, and I would soon be weaned onto white, pasty, refined cereal, then to sweet, crunchy, refined cereal with added sugar, when old enough to add even more sugar by the spoonful. I was a *junk food* addict before the term was originated, and never knew it until it was too late. Neither did my parents, my many doctors, or millions of others around the world who were falling with me into a deep, dark hole of sickness.

We were the baby boomers. Despite increasing life expectancy, we would become less healthy than the previous generation, according to the Centers for Disease Control and Prevention. We would not only be sicker but costlier to the healthcare system as well. And, thanks to junk food, we were destined to form the foundation of an impending *overfat pandemic*.

I was one of the lucky who managed to escape.

Today, people know me as a slim, 160-pound, six-foot person, essentially the same as at high school graduation. But throughout childhood and into adulthood, I was overfat. At times I didn't *appear* to have too much body fat. My metabolism, however, was like an obese person's, eventually experiencing the full spectrum of body fat.

I recall not wanting to step onto the scale anymore after seeing my weight go above 200 pounds. Hitting the other extreme was just as bad, falling to a debilitating underweight state of ninety-six pounds; yet still, there was excess fat—*sarcopenic obesity* is a condition, usually seen in the elderly yet I was only in my early twenties, of muscle-wasting concomitant with surplus body fat.

Needless to say, I bought a lot of clothes during those years to keep up with changes in body composition.

Before age twenty-five, chronic disease made its mark. I had been hospitalized numerous times with severe inflammatory bowel disease (IBD), was diagnosed with type 2 diabetes, and was exhausted and depressed. A few years later, I was diagnosed with fatty liver, another condition usually seen only later in life. To top it all off, learning disabilities made education complicated, while attention deficit disorder (ADD) led to serious social dysfunction.

I was frustrated and looking for answers when, finally, it hit me. I was addicted to junk food, since birth if not before. It kept me on a grave roller coaster ride destined to derail. It would have killed me before age forty. But nature called. I was able to break through to the other side, understanding that *healthy food* was my real medicine. It seemed too simple of a concept, though physically making the change was not easy. But I made it out of desperation.

After all, just *reducing* junk food didn't work. Junk food proved to be the exception to the "everything in moderation" slogan. More precisely, I learned how immediately the body's metabolism was impaired with just a small amount of processed carbohydrate, or even a healthy product with added sugar. I forged ahead to better understand, and eventually the discipline reaped amazing results.

All my conditions disappeared one by one.

Over the next forty years, all the international and national health agencies began warning that the world was getting too overweight and obese. From the National Institutes of Health to the World Health Organization, they eventually began calling it an epidemic. Unfortunately, they did not use the "F" word much. *Fat* was politically incorrect, and some in the public sector even considered it offensive. Instead, most research and published scientific studies nearly ignored the fact that excess body fat was serious—the concern was being overweight and obese.

Instead of acknowledging overfat, people commonly measured weight and body mass index (BMI), a calculation based on weight and height.

A lot of money was spent on counting all the overweight and obese people around the world, emphasizing that no country has ever reduced these rising rates. But they still avoided the issue of body fat, so much that an overfat pandemic exploded over the past four decades with almost no one noticing.

As it turns out, the number of overfat people is much greater than those who are overweight and obese. Yet something important was missing—a remedy. That's what this book is about.

In order to understand the remedy for the overfat pandemic, we must consider our food supply. Though our ancestors knew how to eat, today mega-conglomerate food companies sell highly processed junk food to billions of people by convincing them it's healthy, but it's not. We'll call these companies *Big Sugar* as an industry because they use the same strategy as Big Tobacco—gimmicks, deception, lies, and lobbyists to sell their products like illicit drug traffickers. It's as profitable as the criminal cartels—actually, more. And for a real-life perspective, Big Sugar is more deadly than Big Tobacco.

While rising rates of chronic disease, lower quality of life, and years of dysfunction at the end of the lifespan, not to mention the emergence of genetic mutations, are bad enough, we just have to take a look around to see one obvious problem caused by bad food: the *overfat* pandemic. This book can help you escape it, if you choose. My goal is not to convince you that junk food is bad—there is already a consensus of that among clinicians, scientists, and almost all of the public—but to give you that extra push you probably need to get through to the other side.

Ten Tenets of Overfat:

1. New research shows that up to 76 percent of the world's population is *overfat*, defined as excess body fat sufficient to impair health. Even people who are not overweight or obese can still be overfat.
2. In just a few generations, an *overfat pandemic* has taken over the world. This happened while processed carbohydrate consumption, including added sugars, increased dramatically, and while the consumption of fats has reduced.
3. This paralleled the popularity of low-fat/low-calorie *diets*, leading millions of dieters to weigh in and be frustrated from poor lasting results, and miserable from restricted

eating and hunger. Those who lose weight often gain it back—plus more. But losing weight does not necessarily mean losing body fat, the reason many normal-weight people are *overfat*.

4. The *overfat* condition contributes to poor metabolic health and a reduction in the body's ability to burn stored fat—thus, fat keeps accumulating (regardless of weight), while health deteriorates.

5. *Overfat* as a condition can lead to fatigue, poor sleep, depression, hunger, immune dysfunction, hormone imbalance, sugar addiction, and impaired aging. It can transition to chronic inflammation, high blood fats, hypertension, atherosclerosis, and insulin resistance. It can also lead to cancer, heart disease, Alzheimer's disease, stroke, diabetes, liver disease, and other chronic conditions.

6. In addition to poor food choices, primarily junk food, even the wrong exercise and other lifestyle stressors can further feed the *overfat* pandemic. The good news: you can reverse the problem quickly.

7. Following a *diet* is counter to our natural instincts and is obviously not the answer. While on a diet, the world got *overfat*. Avoiding diets can help us relearn how best to eat for our bodies.

8. Also avoid the bathroom scale—weight is deceptive, and not a measure of body fat. Instead, *waist size* is a better way for most people to monitor body fat—as fat-burning progresses, we get leaner with a smaller waist.

9. This book will help *you* manage your own health, individualize your particular lifestyle needs to burn off more body fat, and reverse the *overfat* trend.

10. You can make the simple, natural lifestyle changes to burn off rather than store excess body fat, get leaner, balance

hormones, be full of energy and brain power, improve health and get more fit, and even be a better athlete.

A word of caution: you might have to buy new clothes sooner than you think.

CHAPTER 1

THE OVERFAT PANDEMIC

New research published January 3, 2017 in the journal *Frontiers of Public Health*[2] suggests that up to 76 percent of the world's population is overfat. While we think of those with excess body fat as overweight or obese, normal-weight adults and children can and are overfat too. In addition, the overfat problem is not only found in inactive people, but many who exercise regularly—even some who are competitive athletes.

I extensively studied this pandemic with my colleagues Professor Paul Laursen and research assistant Ivan Rivera-Dominguez. While I've been referring to the condition of overfat my whole career, we were the first researchers to globally quantify those who are overfat versus overweight and obese, writing that the well-documented obesity epidemic is merely the tip of an overfat iceberg.

Since the number of overfat people was found to be shockingly high, we described the problem as a hidden pandemic that has quietly overtaken the world—one that most people, including the scientific and health-care communities and governmental agencies, seemed to never have noticed. The pandemic may be affecting an astonishing 5.5 billion people—and counting. The number of overfat people is much greater than those who are overweight or obese (see chart).

Condition	Percent of world	Numbers of people
Overweight & Obese	39–49 percent	2.8–3.5 billion
Overfat	62–76 percent	3.5–5.5 billion

The overfat pandemic is truly a global problem. It affects people of all ages and incomes, and in recent years appears significantly in both developed and developing nations. And if you think that up to 76 percent of the population being overfat seems extreme, it's not. In fact, we were conservative in our analysis. Consider the fact that, in developing countries, the *underweight* population, mostly due to malnutrition, skews these numbers, bringing the averages down. If we only look at the Western world, most countries have overfat rates much higher than 76 percent (more on this later).

In our study, we defined the condition of *overfat* as having sufficient excess body fat to impair health. And while obesity has been considered the world's largest preventable health disorder, overfat has now replaced it.

The overfat pandemic poses a global concern because of its strong association with three devastating and expensive factors:

- **Increased disease risk**. The onset of a variety of disease risk factors include the overfat state itself, along with overweight and obesity, high blood cholesterol and triglycerides, hypertension, high blood sugar and pre-diabetes, non-alcoholic fatty liver, polycystic ovary syndrome and infertility, and insulin resistance, to name a few.

- **Rising rates of chronic disease**. High levels of body fat can cause low-grade chronic inflammation, precursors to various downstream diseases, those that most Western people, and many others, will die from, including type 2 diabetes, heart disease, cancer, stroke, Alzheimer's, and many others. These, along with increased disease risks, reduce the quality of life.

- **Escalating health-care costs**. With increasing numbers of health-care problems in more people who are also living longer, skyrocketing health-care costs are ravaging the world economy. Worldwide, chronic diseases are estimated to be responsible for over $17 trillion cumulative economic loss between 2011 and 2030 due to healthcare expenditures, reduced productivity, and lost capital. In the US alone, health-care costs rose to over $3 trillion in 2015.

THE GROWING PANDEMIC

The World Health Organization recently stated that no country has been able to stop the growth of overweight and obese people. Likewise, for the overfat pandemic—it continues throughout the world in developed nations, and is expanding even faster in developing nations. In fact, developing nations are undergoing a *nutrition transition*, in which populations in a single generation are moving from starvation to overfat.

While rates of obesity may be slowing in some Western countries, the overfat pandemic is still growing because normal-weight individuals can still be overfat.

One reason for the explosion of the overfat pandemic over the past forty years, and why it continues with no indication of stopping, is that the pandemic is continuously being fed the very foods that cause people to become overfat. Junk food is cheap and widely available, people are addicted to sugar, governments continue recommending it, and most health-care organizations have not done much to remedy the problem. National survey data in the US, for example, has indicated that during these decades, consumption of refined carbohydrates has increased by up to 900 percent.

This leaves *you*, the individual, to address the problem of managing your health by personalizing the way you eat. That is the focus of this book.

BODY COMPOSITION

In part because the focus has been on weight and not fat for so many years, the paucity of research on precise measures of body fat content has left us without a consensus on what normal levels should be for optimal health. Because scale weight has been the focus, definitions of overweight and obesity are quite precise. The current standard in the clinical setting is through measurement of BMI (defined as an individual's weight in kilograms divided by their height in meters squared). Standard cutoff points for underweight, normal weight, overweight, or obese are as follows:

- <18.5 = underweight
- 18.5–24.9 = normal weight

- 25–29.9 = overweight (also called *pre-obese*)
- >30 = obese

The traditional BMI is not a direct measure of body fat, and is not a precise measure when considering differences in gender, age, and race.

There are varying opinions by scientists about body fat levels. Most cutoff points for percent body fat by governmental and health organizations are associated with obesity levels and not ideal "normal" ranges of body fat. This is frustrating for many people, who are used to stepping on a scale and reading a single number, but body fat measures are more elusive. Even if we could easily measure them, there is still not a consensus for normal ranges of percent body fat.

STAY OFF THE BATHROOM SCALE!

Stepping onto the scale to measure your weight can be misleading. Excess body fat may take up a lot of room on the thighs, belly, and elsewhere, but it really doesn't weigh very much. Body weight does not necessarily reflect body fat.

While most people consider excess body weight and body fat as synonymous, it's simply untrue. As a weight-conscious society, for many people stepping onto the scale each morning is a powerful ritual—and one that's difficult to break.

The scale is more so a measure of water, especially found in muscles, rather than a measure of fat. However, body fat takes up much more space than muscle and water do. In fact, some patients I helped lose significant amounts of body fat actually didn't lose much scale weight—some actually gained weight while trimming inches of fat off their waists! With exercise that helps lead to fat loss, there is often a small amount of muscle development, which adds weight, sometimes offsetting the relatively small amount of scale weight lost from fat.

The fitness market is full of devices that claim to accurately measure body fat. Most are not very accurate, though. Underwater (hydrostatic) weighing and DEXA (dual-energy X-ray absorptiometry) scan, also used to measure bone density, are two of the best, and correlate well with waist circumference (discussed later). However, they are not often practical and accessible, and usually costly considering that more than one test is needed to compare progress. There are also formulas based on BMI, gender, age, and other factors that have value too, but also are not as practical.

One reason why measuring percent body fat accurately is not an easy task is that we are all individuals with variations that have to be taken into account but often cannot. So it's important to focus only on yourself and not make comparisons to some "normal" ranges that don't really exist, or certain other people or periods in your past when body fat levels appeared lower. Monitoring your personal progress is best done with a simple measure of your waist.

WHY "OVERFAT"?

In the context of health and related body fat levels the use of the term *overfat* is quite acceptable throughout the healthcare world. And now, especially with published research demonstrating that overfat is also found in those who are of normal weight or BMI, it could become accepted by virtually all people. It's important to logically embrace any health issue, especially one that causes so much of the world's illness.

The overfat study brings to light the fact that new terminology—specifically the term *overfat*—is important to replace the old notions of *overweight* and *obese*. Better, more clinically descriptive, terms can significantly help those in health care and the public address the problem of excess body fat by using the term overfat, as opposed to obesity and overweight. It may also be more helpful moving forward in addressing this global pandemic.

UNDERFAT AND NORMAL FAT

In addition to the number of overfat people, the study also estimated 9 to 10 percent of the world population may be *underfat*. While we think of the condition of underfat as being due to starvation, the number of people starving worldwide is actually rapidly dropping. However, an aging population, an increase in chronic disease, and a rising number of excessive exercisers—those with *anorexia athletica*—are adding to the number of non-starving underfat individuals. Having too little body fat can also impair health.

While the number of people who exercise is growing worldwide, ranging from those who do minimal training to triathletes, marathoners, and others who compete seriously, clearly more are falling into the overfat and underfat categories as well.

This leaves as little as 14 percent of the world's general population with normal body-fat percentages. Unfortunately, only some unknown portion of the 14 percent are healthy individuals.

IN SHORT: WHY IS THE WORLD OVERFAT?

Before we go further into the various issues of overfat, I want to briefly answer this important question because too much of the world is basically misinformed about it.

Overconsumption of food and reduced physical activity are the two most commonly discussed reasons for the overfat pandemic. It's the current scientific consensus. While many clinicians, scientists, health-care agencies, and others claim that excess calories and lack of exercise are to blame, the major issue is that the focus is on merely treating symptoms and not addressing the cause of the overfat pandemic. This is part of the problem, and to a large degree, is a key reason the pandemic is still growing. When carefully questioning this common equation, we uncover a more primary, more important *cause* of the overfat pandemic—refined carbohydrate consumption, the primary ingredient of junk food.

Most meals consumed throughout the world include junk food ingredients, typically added sugars and/or refined flour (which quickly converts to sugar after eating it). The intake of junk food has been rising for generations. Here's how it happens:

Consuming refined carbohydrates causes people to be hungrier, and crave sugar, with the result of eating more junk food. It's not hunger from a lack of food, but from a lack of healthy, nutrient-rich food, all triggering metabolic impairments in the form of hormone imbalances and reducing the body's ability to burn body fat for energy. The result is that we keep storing fat.

In addition to sugar cravings, the hunger results in fatigue and is another common symptom of eating junk food. People who are more fatigued exercise less and even move less over the course of the day. Taking the elevator rather than the stairs (even to the first floor), driving around the parking lot waiting for a space closer to where they're going, and other habits have become popular.

When consumed, refined carbohydrates, such as products made from flour—including bread, bagels, cereals, and all those snack foods—not only turn to sugar. Most also contain *added* sugars—a double whammy. No surprise that sugar addiction is what keeps most people stuck in this vicious cycle. Like Big Tobacco, Big Sugar wants to keep their customers.

This vicious cycle leads to a condition called *overfat*.

While most people *think* they know what junk food is, many have been fooled. In truth, there is an even more dangerous line of products out there capable of actually allowing the overfat pandemic to grow even more: the *new* junk food, deceptively disguised throughout our food supply.

FIXING OVERFAT

The overfat pandemic *was* preventable decades ago. It *is* preventable in its ongoing pattern of growth. Now we know that it's also reversible. This can be accomplished with three key suggestions that will be defined, emphasized, explored, and discussed throughout the book, making the process of self-health management an easier one for you:

1. Stop eating junk food.
2. Determine your level of carbohydrate intolerance.
3. Adjust your eating to changes in carbohydrate intolerance that occurs with age.

Next, let's see who is most vulnerable to being overfat.

CHAPTER 2

WHO IS OVERFAT?

It's easy to observe the high numbers of overfat people. Just look around while out shopping, at the gym, at a social event, or elsewhere. The overfat pandemic affects people of all incomes, both genders, in all areas of the world, and of all races and ages. Below I have outlined a variety of groups of people who are usually overfat.

OVERWEIGHT AND OBESE ADULTS

Most people who are overweight and obese are also overfat. The number of adults who are overweight and obese includes up to 49 percent of the world population. This may sound like a large number, but it's actually misleading and on the low side because it also considers many people in developing nations who are malnourished and underfat. A look at only

Western countries where the underfat population is very low shows an even bleaker picture of overfat. Countries like the US have rates of overweight and obese at 70 percent, meaning that overfat rates are much higher than the global rate of 76 percent shown in the research, as shown below.

THE NORMAL-WEIGHT OVERFAT

In addition to those who are overweight and obese, many people who are normal weight are still overfat. They include those who are called *metabolically obese, normal weight*, which is a condition that affects 20 to 22 percent or more of normal-weight adults and children.

These individuals have sufficient excess stores of body fat to impair health. This condition includes people with excess fat deposits in or around organs such as the liver, heart, and muscles. While this tends to occur with aging, the problem is now seen in younger people as well.

Another group of individuals with excess body fat who are not overweight or obese are those with *sarcopenic obesity*. This health condition occurs more typically later in life, although it sometimes occurs in younger people with debilitating conditions. Sarcopenia is a common problem with aging, resulting from a loss of muscle mass and strength. But along with reduced muscle mass there could be an infiltration of excess body fat.

OVERWEIGHT AND OBESE CHILDREN

As a group, children who are overweight or obese are a fast-growing segment of the overfat pandemic. In most cases, if they don't adopt healthy eating habits, they are more likely to

SOME OF THE HIGHEST OVERFAT COUNTRIES

In the US, New Zealand, Greece, and Iceland, about 50 percent of children are overfat. Below are the estimated average percentages of the highest overweight/obese and overfat adults in some countries.

Country	Overweight & Obese	Overfat
US	70 percent	91 percent
Iceland	67 percent	87 percent
New Zealand	66 percent	86 percent
UK	62 percent	82 percent
Australia	62 percent	82 percent
Greece	61 percent	81 percent

become overfat adults. This has created an even more serious problem because children are now developing adult diseases. Close to 30 percent of the children in the US are overweight or obese, a similar percentage as that of other Western nations, with the number of overfat children now over 50 percent.

PEOPLE WITH EXCESS BELLY FAT

Too much belly fat is bad. Also referred to as abdominal or central obesity, more than 30 percent of normal-weight adults and children have too much belly fat. Since it can occur in normal-weight non-obese people, a better term would be *abdominal overfat*, or ab fat. This problem contributes significantly to the overfat population.

Abdominal overfat is particularly bad because, more than higher levels of body fat elsewhere, this metabolically active fat depot has a potentially greater negative impact on health, regardless of the person's weight. Waist circumference has a direct correlation with the risk of developing heart disease, stroke, type 2 diabetes, hypertension, cancer, and other chronic diseases, in addition to its relationship to the overfat state.

Excess ab fat is built up in large part because refined carbohydrates, through the mechanism of insulin production by the pancreas, triggers the movement of fat stores in the body's periphery, from thighs and arms, for example, where it is less harmful, to abdominal deposits, where it's most harmful.

While those who are overweight, obese, and have sarcopenic obesity have increased risk for disease, those who are normal weight but have increased belly fat can be even more unhealthy or have higher risk of disease, including higher mortality rates.

Moreover, those with excess belly fat are the fastest-growing segment of the overfat pandemic.

MEASURING OVERFAT

Quantifying belly fat is easy, by measuring our waist. Waist circumference may be a more practical and superior solution than using the bathroom scale or BMI for identification of one's overfat state. Most important is that monthly monitoring can provide information about trends—is your waist getting smaller and therefore you're progressing; is it getting larger; are you remaining the same?

Over the years, various forms of waist measurements have been used, but the best current one is the waist-to-height ratio (WHtR). This is accurate for adults and children of both genders around the world. While it doesn't indicate percentage of body fat, for which there is no scientific consensus of normal and abnormal, a WHtR of .50 and above measured at the level of the belly button (umbilicus) indicates being overfat, defined as an excess amount of body fat to impair health. For example:

- A person with a 30-inch waist and height of 62 inches: WHtR = .48; normal fat.
- A person with a 36-inch waist and height of 70 inches: WHtR = .51; overfat.
- The key message is simple: *Our waist circumference should be less than half our height.*

HOW TO MEASURE YOUR WAIST

1. First, get a flexible tape, but not one that stretches.
2. Wrap the tape around your waist, directly on the skin and not over clothes, at the level of the belly button, keeping the tape horizontal (doing it in front of a mirror can help with this).
3. Hold the tape snug, but don't compress the skin too tight.
4. Relax your belly, and stand up straight with both feet on the floor.
5. Note the measurement in inches or centimeters.
6. Keep a record of your measurements.

Avoid the obsession of measuring every day or even weekly, which can only contribute to emotional stress (and stress can actually impair the process of fat loss). Too frequent measurements are not sensitive enough to reflect minor changes. Instead, measure your waist once a month on the same day and time (in the morning before breakfast works well).

Most people will already know if they have gained or lost body fat because their pants fit too tightly or loosely. In addition, if you lost body fat, other people may ask if you're losing weight. This is because a slight amount of fat loss in the face makes you look thinner, and people recognize that and mistake this for weight loss. (Reductions in body fat are not always associated with weight loss.)

The rapid rise in abdominal overfat has negated some studies that show a leveling off of overweight prevalence and/or obesity. But during the period from 2000–2014, US adult waist sizes have increased significantly. As reported by the Centers for Disease Control and Prevention, US men average a waist circumference of almost 40 inches, and women 37.5 inches.

EXERCISE AND OVERFAT

Surprisingly, those who exercise are not necessarily spared from the overfat pandemic. One might think that exercise is an important way to prevent or correct the overfat condition. While this could be the case, too often it's not, as indicated by the many people who run marathons, perform triathlons, and regularly workout—activities that burn a lot of calories—yet many are still overfat.

One reason for this is that many people burn a lot of sugar calories, but not enough fat calories. Certainly exercise burns a higher amount of calories than when we are inactive. So ask yourself, which calories are you burning more of?

Exercise has many important benefits, including the potential to help the body burn more fat.

Understanding what you are eating is even more important for preventing and correcting the overfat condition. Many people who exercise eat too much junk food, and often purposely consume more sugar, believing they need the energy. But fat-burning provides more energy for active people. An important introduction about the cause of the overfat pandemic was discussed in chapter 1, and is worth repeating here:

Consuming refined carbohydrates causes people to be hungrier, and crave sugar, with the result of eating more junk food. It's not hunger from a lack of food, but from a lack of healthy, nutrient-rich food, all triggering metabolic impairments in the form of hormone imbalances and reducing the body's ability to burn body fat for energy. The result is that we keep storing fat.

While eating nutritious foods is a more important way to stimulate our metabolism to burn more fat calories, exercise can help the process. But many people who work out eat the wrong foods and exercise in ways that burn more sugar calories and not enough fat. In a person with a healthy metabolism, even high-intensity training burns a surprising amount of fat.

Whether you're training to run a marathon, working out on a stationary bike, doing weight lifting or any other activity, it does not guarantee that you will rid the body of excess fat. In fact, sometimes people increase their body fat levels.

The important part of this discussion is that those who exercise are not immune to being overfat. This issue—and how to remedy the problem—is detailed in chapter 8.

Looking at all the possible reasons for being overfat and the populations most affected are not as important as taking a look at *yourself* and understanding your own particular needs and what to do about it. As I've emphasized previously, the food we eat plays a primary role.

CHAPTER 3

WHY THE WORLD IS OVERFAT

After discussing the overfat pandemic and knowing who might fit that definition, it's time to start getting into the details of why the world is overfat and how you can manage the process of reducing excess body fat to get healthy and fit.

For decades, a variety of health practitioners have helped many people switch from a junk food diet to healthy eating, although this approach was not always in vogue. I've done the same my entire career. Despite our successes, we were ridiculed for not following the trends of unhealthy food recommendations that included high amounts of refined carbohydrates and low-fat snacks. Don't be swayed by thinking "low-fat" means healthy; it usually means high sugar, half of which can turn to fat and be stored.

Today, scientists know the reasons why junk food makes people overfat. Some have been publishing this information for a long time (see the bibliography). This has prompted Big Sugar to change their strategy, to promote more healthy-appearing foods they call natural, whole grain, or otherwise nourishing, yet almost all of it is junk food.

I don't want to waste pages describing the studies and science behind all the good and bad foods out there—essentially trying to convince you to avoid the bad and eat the good ones. Instead, I want to help you succeed by managing your own health—you'll quickly learn which food to avoid and how the facts of food, including the long-standing misinformation campaigns by Big Sugar and even governments, health-care professionals, and others. These problems have contributed to the cause of the overfat pandemic for decades. And it's why the world continues getting more overfat.

TWO INTERNATIONAL CUISINES

It's really quite simple—there are two distinct cuisines in the world today, two kinds of foods:

- *Healthy food.* It's real, naturally occurring, unadulterated and unprocessed, and nutrient-rich. If you can grow or raise it, it's real. Included are fresh fruits and vegetables, lentils and beans, eggs, real cheese, whole pieces of meat (such as fish, beef, chicken), nuts, seeds, and similar items. Consuming these foods provides a great potential for both immediate and long-term health benefits because they are dense in nutrients and do no harm. They are also delicious.
- *Junk food* is everything else. If you have to ask what junk food is, you're probably eating it. Lacking nutrients, addicting, quickly converting to stored fat are

all characteristics of junk food, which is harmful to everyone. And we get addicted to it easily, in part because it keeps making us hungry for more junk food. These items are processed, manufactured, and have added chemicals, sugars, and other unhealthy ingredients that can adversely affect both short-term and long-term health. Most importantly, they replace healthy foods in our diets. We all know about fast food, soda, the many products with added sugars, and other junk foods, but Big Sugar continually reinvents junk food to create new forms that *appear* healthy but are not. They do such a good job disguising junk food that most people, despite knowing that junk food is bad food, buy it. Traditional junk foods include those based on sugar and refined flour, and are the primary cause of the overfat pandemic. Not just candy, cookies, chips, and fast food, but items once considered healthy, such as yogurt that's typically high in sugar, canned fruit in sugar-syrup, processed vegetables (canned, frozen, or from fast-food outlets) with sugar, processed wheat, corn and other flour, baked beans in a sugar and starch sauce, processed cheese and cheese spreads, cold cuts (bologna, salami, chicken, and turkey loaf) fish sticks (which usually contain sugar), peanut butter (typically containing sugar and trans fat), and thousands of others in grocery stores, markets, even health stores, and retail outlets often fall into the "bad-for-you" category. Always read the ingredients.

Because junk food is so harmful, some health authorities want to refer to junk food as *pathogenic food*. This name refers to the foods' capability to cause pathological conditions, including the overfat pandemic. But spreading this new designation won't happen soon enough, thanks to the ongoing multimillion-dollar marketing campaigns waged by Big Sugar.

Big Sugar's main product category is junk food, and is one of the most successful business ventures on the planet, even greater than Big Tobacco, only more deceptive. Large amounts of it are in almost all households worldwide, and even widespread in the developing world, where in only one generation, millions of starving people have now become overfat, thanks to junk food.

It's widely believed that the phrase *junk food* was coined in 1972 by Michael Jacobson, director of the American Center for Science in the Public Interest (a consumer advocacy organization that focuses on health and nutrition). But defining junk food has been a difficult task, partly because the number of items it represents is alarmingly high, and also because the food landscape is always changing with so-called new and improved products coming and going almost daily.

THE *NEW* JUNK FOOD

It's everywhere. The new junk food is front and center in our homes and workplaces, schools, restaurants (even the fancy ones), in takeout and deli counters, in all grocery stores, and even in health food stores. We celebrate life with junk food, rationalizing the consumption of it as moderation, but in fact more people consume large amounts of it. We think we know what it is and how to avoid it, but it's no longer that easy.

Self-conscious eaters have become so accustomed to going into a grocery store, deli, or takeout or fast-food restaurant *believing* there are healthy choices. Or we shop for healthy ingredients to prepare food at home, *thinking* we're avoiding junk food. You may have even learned to avoid the fast-food restaurants and baking or cereal aisles of grocery stores that are filled with sugar and refined flour, and are buying these from health stores instead. But this belief is the result of Big Sugar's long-standing creative marketing campaigns, as they are also well-represented in health food stores. They have successfully repackaged junk food to create a new and improved image.

Most junk food is made of sugar and/or refined flours. In addition to their use as ingredients, these two items continue to be a staple in pantries and counters of most homes, and have for generations.

Whole grain junk food has been the big bandwagon for decades, even promoted by governments claiming we should eat more of it. But it's a primary reason the overfat pandemic continues. The whole grain disguise has been with us for generations in various forms and names.

But all these so-called whole grain products are highly refined. True whole grains are not easy to find, and most people won't eat them because they don't have the *mouth feel* or sweetness of junk food. Highly refined wheat flours, basically the same as yesterday's *white flour*, is the norm. It's often colored, highly processed, and labeled to appear like the natural version but outsells real whole grains more than ten to one in the West.

Most consumers have never seen wheat berries, the raw kernel used to make flour. Many have also never seen other grains, such as whole oatmeal. A clue that they are real has to do with cook time. For example, real oats take 45 minutes or more to prepare. Compare this to junk food oats, which may take one minute to cook or less, as some only require adding hot water.

Despite what the label says, virtually all other ready-to-eat breakfast items are junk food too, with most containing added sugars.

Most certified organic items are junk too. In fact, *organic junk food* continues to be one of the fastest-growing segments of the natural foods industry. It leads the line of new junk food. Organic sugar, refined flour, and other junk food is just as harmful to our bodies while costing more.

JUNK FOOD FRUITS AND VEGGIES?

While food scientists have created new junk food to fool consumers, other agriculture scientists have done something very similar to natural foods. Knowing there's a growing sweet tooth that makes people choose sweeter fruits and vegetables, they have manipulated many plant foods to grow them with more sugar and starch (which turns to sugar). Apples, peaches, tomatoes, squashes, and most others are bigger than ever, sometimes two to three times the size of food our grandparents ate, and with higher amounts of sugar. Yes, it's natural sugar, but it still can quickly contribute to carbohydrate intolerance in many people. The worst ones include:

Grapes	All potatoes
Bananas	Yams
Pineapple	Corn
Watermelon	Parsnips
Dates	Pumpkin

In addition, dried fruits, including raisins, are a very concentrated sweet food, so avoid them along with concentrated items like ketchup (which usually has added sugar as well).

Of course, most so-called energy bars are junk food too. They are really *fatigue bars* because they zap our energy (right after you get that short-lived sugar rush). Likewise for sports drinks and other liquid beverages claiming to be healthy.

Virtually all liquid drinks, except for pure water, are junk food. In particular, avoid fruit *juices,* as they are a highly concentrated food, which is metabolized like refined carbohydrates. Most sports drinks are also high in refined sugar.

In addition, most "diet" products are junk foods. Low-fat, low-calorie products are still popular, even though they can contribute significantly to the overfat pandemic. Most contain sugar and refined flour. Included are diet sodas (see Artificial Sweeteners, below).

The glycemic index is a measure of how much insulin is released after consuming a particular carbohydrate. Some people use this as an eating guide and it's also a part of many diet programs. Unfortunately, most foods on the glycemic index are junk food. People following this approach have learned the *glycemic game*—add protein, fat, and/or fiber to carbohydrate

ARTIFICIAL SWEETENERS

Just the name tells you it's junk food. The new junk food fake sugars, or low-calorie sweeteners, are no longer called artificial. But studies show that those consuming low-calorie or fake sugars are more overfat than those who don't consume them, leading especially to increases in belly fat.

Alcohol sugars are the latest trend. While they don't have many calories, these chemicals are not healthy. They are popular selling ingredients, and often added to other junk food products so they could be called low-cal, low-carb, or zero-carb. Diet soda is among the more popular of these products. They are unhealthy because they contribute to maintaining your sweet tooth, while tricking the brain to store more body fat.

The most natural non-caloric sweetener, stevia, is usually highly processed, although the plant itself is quite natural. However, the sweet taste is still the problem. Getting rid of your sweet tooth is an important part of the process of getting healthy and burning more body fat.

foods or meals to reduce the glycemic index, thinking it's now a healthy food. It still does not change the amount of carbohydrate consumed, especially when it's junk food.

Reading a food's ingredient list can often tell you about added sugars, cornstarch, flour, and hard-to-pronounce chemicals. But if a product even has an ingredient list, you might think twice about eating it. Ingredient lists are not always available in a restaurant, deli, or other eateries. When in doubt, avoid it.

For those on the go, junk food is synonymous with fast food, and includes most meat, fish, and veggie burgers, fries, pizza, fried chicken, and items that are battered, coated, or have sauces. Like junk food itself, fast-food restaurants have changed their look to appear more natural and wholesome, but sell just junk food. Likewise for company, school, hospital, and other cafeterias, which serve prepared foods with significant amounts of sugar and other refined carbohydrates. Most international foods are not exempt from the junk food category. This includes Asian foods (high in sugar, starch, and/or flour), especially sushi rice (added sugar), sweetened pickles and teriyaki, Italian foods (tomato sauce typically has moderate amounts of sugar), and many foods today are prepared with a crust or coating of flour.

Even high-end restaurants, while having healthy options, still also offer a lot of fancy junk foods made with sugar and refined flour.

Going to a deli for lunch? The popular ham and American cheese on a roll is all junk food. Most sliced deli meats contain sugar. Tuna, chicken, and egg salads usually have sugar, and even a plain vegetable salad with low-cal dressing contains sugar, as do croutons. Virtually all pasta, noodles, and similar items are junk food, as are bagels and rice cakes.

How much junk food causes harm? That depends on how carbohydrate intolerant you have become. One bite can be enough for some people, especially those addicted to sugar. Certainly a junk food snack or meal can significantly alter one's physiology in a negative way, storing more body fat and reducing our ability to burn it for energy.

By now you might be asking, what *can* I eat? Without junk food there are still plenty of healthy options for delicious meals, snacks, and even desserts. Today, it's much easier to find healthy food that's ready to eat, and shopping for healthy ingredients to prepare great meals at home is easy too. Depending on your particular needs—how much natural carbohydrate you must limit—there are many options. These include most vegetables and fruits, eggs, cheeses, meats, lentils, honey, cocoa, and many others.

Fortunately, we are now seeing stores and restaurants that cater to people with the desire to avoid junk food. If you look carefully, you'll find items made from real foods without junk food ingredients: a leaf lettuce salad with tomatoes, red peppers, carrots, and slices of real roast beef or Swiss cheese. Hold the mayo and ketchup, but mustard or sour cream (depending on the ingredients) or olive oil and vinegar would be OK. A stir-fry of fish and vegetables cooked in butter or coconut oil could work too. Coffee, tea, and water may be the only drink options. Just be careful, as most of the establishments—as "natural" and "healthy" as they appear—also serve junk food. Otherwise, they would not stay in business.

Humans don't tolerate large amounts of natural carbohydrates. Our ancestors never consumed even moderate amounts as they evolved primarily on fatty meats, including fish, and vegetables. Today, after only a few thousand years of increasing intakes of carbohydrates, and for only a few

HOW CARBOHYDRATES MAKE YOU OVERFAT

A decades-long myth promoted by Big Sugar—in bed with the weight-loss industry—is the low-fat/high-carbohydrate approach. They promote the myth that fat is bad because it increases body fat, and therefore eating low-fat carbohydrates—sugar—should be the emphasis on weight control. But that's not how our bodies work, and the result has been increased refined carbohydrate consumption, lower fat consumption, and an overfat pandemic.

FAT STORAGE

It's a metabolic mechanism developed by humans millions of years ago. It was a way to assure we had enough stored energy, or fat, during times of low food availability. While too much fat and protein can increase fat stores, carbohydrates convert to fat for storage too, and at the same time tend to keep it stored. This has to do with insulin.

In a healthy body, the hormone insulin, produced in the pancreas when we eat carbohydrates (and very large amounts of protein), has a number of actions:

- About half the carbohydrates you eat are used by muscles for energy.
- A small amount (up to 10 percent) is stored as sugar (glycogen).
- Forty to 50 percent percent of the carbs you eat turn to fat and are stored.
- Increases the use of sugar for energy and reduces fat-burning.
- Moves more body fat stores into the belly.

Too much carbohydrate consumption could increase the production of insulin, leading to more carbohydrate foods being converted to stored fat, less fat-burning, more belly fat, and being overfat.

Consuming too much refined carbs earlier in life can lead to insulin resistance and insulin overproduction. In many people this can lead to insulin levels suddenly falling significantly (due to "exhaustion" of the pancreatic cells that produce it), leading to type 2 diabetes.

generations, refined carbohydrates are a modern "staple" that those who are overfat (and even those who aren't) tolerate much less. In short, we don't tolerate refined carbohydrates. Eating them damages our metabolism and increases stored body fat, making us intolerant to those carbohydrates. They should be avoided.

Natural carbohydrate foods can be very healthy, and may not adversely affect your metabolism like junk food. However, it's important to find the amount that's best for you, and not exceed this amount. This has to do with your level of *carbohydrate intolerance* or CI.

WHAT IS CARBOHYDRATE INTOLERANCE?

Health-care agencies, politicians, researchers, and others have made quite a mess out of something so simple as food. Big Sugar has made sure of that, encouraging governmental dietary recommendations that promote junk food to the world as healthy. The result has caused billions of people to become intolerant to carbohydrates. It's why there is an overfat pandemic.

You can change that by managing your health and choosing the foods best for your body's needs. The first step is finding how much natural carbohydrate you can tolerate and don't exceed it. An increased carbohydrate intolerance, also called CI, can trigger three metabolic problems:

- Low-grade body-wide chronic inflammation, a very early and asymptomatic start of the disease process.
- Insulin resistance and the over-production of insulin. This is an early stage of diabetes called prediabetes, along with other dysfunction (often combined into

the metabolic syndrome). The dysregulation of insulin reduces fat-burning.

- Storing more body fat. Insulin also converts more of the carbohydrate consumed into fat (sometimes up to 50 percent of it), increases belly fat, disrupts hormone balance, and creates a variety of signs and symptoms listed below.

SIGNS AND SYMPTOMS OF CI: TAKE THE SURVEY

These are questions I asked patients to help evaluate the risk or existence of CI. Answer "yes" or "no" to these questions:

- Poor concentration or sleepiness after meals?
- Increased intestinal gas or bloating after meals?
- Frequently hungry?
- Increasing abdominal fat or facial fat (especially cheeks)?
- Frequently fatigued or low energy?
- Insomnia or sleep apnea?
- Waist size increasing with age?
- Fingers swollen/feeling "tight" after exercise?
- Personal or family history of diabetes, kidney stones or gallstones, gout, high blood pressure, high LDL cholesterol or triglycerides, heart disease, stroke, or cancer?
- Low meat, fish, or egg intake?
- Frequent cravings for sweets or caffeine?
- Polycystic ovary (ovarian cysts) or infertility for women?

Those answering "yes" to more than two may have an increased risk for CI.

In addition to the signs and symptoms above, some other possible problems associated with CI range from physical and biochemical conditions, to mental-emotional ones, including:

- Chronic pain
- High LDL cholesterol and triglycerides

- Liver dysfunction
- Arthritis
- Pre-hypertension/hypertension
- Gout
- Kidney stones
- Gallstones
- Pre-diabetes and diabetes
- Osteoporosis
- Hormone imbalance in men and women

There is also a wide spectrum of brain dysfunction associated with CI that includes various mental and emotional conditions. These range from cognitive dysfunction, including poor memory and Alzheimer's disease, depression, anxiety, and others.

WHAT TO DO

If all this sounds complicated and difficult to manage, it's really not. We've become so used to being told what to eat by so-called health authorities and being influenced by advertising, and not managing our own health, that we forget we live in a world where junk food reigns and being aware of it has to be front and center for our brain. So the first of three key factors outlined in this book is this:

1. Stop eating all junk food.
For some, this is easier said than done because sugar addiction is real and keeps us craving and eating it, until we rid the brain and body of it.

When in doubt about a certain food, avoid it. An important consideration is this: as you eliminate junk food you must add healthy food into your meals to avoid a caloric deficit. In particular, include healthy fats like coconut and olive oils, butter or ghee, along with a lot of vegetables except for corn and potatoes. An important guide is hunger.

THE "H" FACTOR: HUNGER

Another reason the world is overfat is hunger, but not for a lack of food. Junk food makes us hungrier, especially for more junk food.

At one time, hearing the word hunger would bring images of malnourished, starving people. This problem still exists, and as starvation has continually been reduced in recent decades, the overfat pandemic rapidly grew. With it came a different kind of malnutrition.

Today, the number of obese people far outweighs those who are starving. And the numbers of people with a *new hunger* has grown too—one frequently felt by *billions* of people. It's a symptom caused not from a lack of food, but from overeating refined carbohydrates, junk food that starves our body's cells of proper nutrients.

Eating healthy food should reduce hunger for hours, while helping you cut excess body fat. But if hunger appears too often, too soon after eating, between meals, or during the night, it can be a problem. It may be indicative that the brain is confused—while it's saying "eat" because the body is starving for fuel, you probably ate not that long ago. This is one of the problems associated with eating sugar and other refined carbohydrates—it affects hormones that ultimately cause hunger.

Protein and fat in the diet can help hunger too, especially in relation to burning off body fat. Studies show that meat-based diets containing 25 to 30 percent protein can result in significant weight loss. Another study demonstrated that 20 grams of supplemental whey protein taken three

HUNGER HORMONES

Produced in the stomach, *ghrelin* is a major hormone that leads us to feel hunger, with levels elevating after periods of an empty stomach. Ghrelin is significantly increased or decreased, along with hunger and the lack of it, by the macronutrients we eat—carbohydrates, proteins, and fats. The hunger hormone is reduced with more fat and protein in the meal, and increased with more carbohydrates.

Those with more body fat have higher amounts of the hunger hormone, with lower levels of those that produce satiety.

Satiation is the feeling of satisfaction or fullness, leading to reduced hunger. This is the result of numerous other gut hormones, including those from the pancreas, along with leptin from stored fat. All are released after a healthy meal.

Carbohydrate intake releases another important hormone that controls hunger—insulin. The more refined the carbohydrate food, the more insulin is released. The result is that more of the carbohydrate consumed turns to fat and is stored. Insulin also reduces the body's ability to burn stored body fat for energy.

times daily significantly helped exercising individuals lose weight and body fat.

Fat in food helps lead to the satisfying feeling after meals. This includes the natural fats in meat, fish, eggs, and other foods, along with butter and ghee, olive oil, and coconut oil. It may simply be that fat reduces hunger by keeping food in the stomach longer.

Fat is also the tastiest of macronutrients. Taste plays an important role in controlling hunger too. Those who don't taste their food well have more hunger hormones.

- The feeling of hunger comes from both the brain and gut.
- The muscles in the stomach that distend and squeeze food out into the small intestines can trigger hunger.

Just the thought of food, including seeing, smelling, or hearing it cook, starts an avalanche of various hormones that regulate hunger. Mental or emotional stress can control hunger too. Companies take advantage of all these factors to entice you to buy and eat.

Other factors associated with hunger include:

- Chewing, which plays an important role in balancing hormones that control hunger. Essentially, the increased number of chews in each bite can reduce hunger.
- How we eat is important too. Eating quickly is associated with reduced satiety and increased body weight, while eating slower has been shown to favor burning off more body fat.
- The time of day when meals are eaten is important. Eating at a time when our internal circadian clock promotes sleep—starting in the early evening and through the night—can add to stored body fat. If we're hungry all evening or wake up during the night hungry, obviously hunger balance is disturbed.
- Aerobic exercise, detailed later, can help balance hunger and satiety hormones because this type of workout is associated with increased fat-burning. But if you are ravenous after a workout, it may be that it's not aerobic, but anaerobic, and promoting less burning of fat calories.
- Hunger is an important symptom to monitor on our journey to burn and keep off excess body fat—it can help guide us to make the most appropriate lifestyle changes that lead to better health. Controlling hunger by avoiding sugar and other refined carbohydrates is an important goal if we want to burn off more body fat.

CHAPTER 4

FAT-BURNING

Body fat serves many important purposes. Without healthy body fat, we would die. Humans have relied on stored body fat wisely for millions of years to evolve successfully. We also oxidize, or burn, body fat for energy. Unfortunately, those who don't burn sufficient body fat accumulate it and can become overfat. In addition, this can literally make our body fat cells sick, contributing to poor health.

FAT-BURNING

The concept of fat-burning is important because stored fat is a great *potential* source of energy for everyday activity. In fact, even a lean person has enough body fat stores worth of energy to walk about 600 miles. People who burn more fat for energy—convert stored body fat to fuel—are usually healthier, energetic, and leaner.

Fat-burning is what happens with a heathy metabolism. It's a vital part of how we obtain our moment-to-moment energy needs.

For generations, people have been told that humans are glucose-based animals, that we are dependent upon sugar for energy. We even learn it in school. It's how *energy bars* got its name. We grab something sweet when busy to keep up with work, when missing a meal, or when hungry; it's used during meetings and conferences, as bowls of candy are placed everywhere. Unfortunately, this idea is not only wrong, but the short-term blip of energy obtained from eating sugar leads to a long-term loss of energy and increased stored body fat, while disabling our ability to burn body fat.

While we certainly use some glucose for energy, without burning fat for fuel we would run out of sugar in a matter of minutes. Sugar is a short-term energy supply, and if we're relying on a lot of it we typically store more body fat since we're using less of it. Fat, on the other hand, is our long-term energy source, and burning more prevents excess storage of it.

Normally, we use a mix of three sources of energy to fuel our body and brain: sugar, fat, and ketones. But if our metabolism is unhealthy, such as when we're carbohydrate intolerant, we burn less fat and ketones, and instead burn more sugar. When we don't burn as much fat, we store it.

Our metabolism regulates how much of each fuel is used, with the quality of food we eat quickly influencing it. Per the graphic below on one end of the spectrum we use high amounts of sugar for energy with low amounts of fat and ketones—this is associated with the overfat condition, fatigued with overall poor health. On the other end, we use

The Fat-Burning Spectrum		
LOW FAT-BURNING————————————➤HIGH FAT-BURNING		
FOOD INTAKE		
High-carbohydrate	Moderate-carbohydrate	Very low-carbohydrate
↓	↓	↓
METABOLISM		
Very low fat-burning	Moderate fat-burning	High fat-burning
Very low ketones	Moderate ketones	High ketones
High sugar-burning	Moderate sugar-burning	Low sugar-burning
↓	↓	↓
HEALTH/FITNESS		
Low health/fitness	Average health/fitness	High health/fitness
High hunger; low energy	Average hunger & energy	Low hunger; high energy
↓	↓	↓
BODY FAT		
Overfat	Average body fat	Healthy body fat

high amounts of fat and ketones for energy with low amounts of sugar—this allows more fat-burning, reduced body fat, increased energy, and improved health.

High fat-burning and high energy go together. Energy is vital for our quality of life, and a better metabolism that burns more fat creates a higher quality of life on many levels. Generating enough energy necessary to supply all the body's needs 24/7 is important—not just during work or exercise, but during play, for better brain function, and even during sleep. This energy comes from carbohydrate, protein, and fat, and is represented as *calories*. We can get more than twice the energy from fat.

Thus, we want to burn more fat calories (which usually increases the use of ketones too) with reducing reliance on sugar calories—this is how our ancestors did it, and how our bodies evolved. A primary way to address the overfat pandemic is to adjust our food intake to burn more fat calories.

MEASURING FAT-BURNING

Very accurate testing of our fat- and sugar-burning "mix"—how much of each we use for energy—is a relatively easy evaluation in a laboratory or clinical environment. This is commonly done during exercise (or metabolic) testing on a treadmill or other stationary device, but it can also be performed at rest. (Measuring ketones are not performed in the same manner, and is described later.)

Called RER (*respiratory exchange ratio*), the test for fat- and sugar-burning relies on the evaluation of oxygen and carbon dioxide to determine the precise measure of how much fat and sugar the body is *oxidizing*, or burning, for energy. A person's RER can help predict and measure a wide variety of health problems, including diabetes, cardiovascular disease, other features of the metabolic syndrome, and the current or future state of being overfat. It also provides information about lean muscle mass, the location at which most of this fat- and sugar-burning takes place.

The RER ranges from 0.7 (100 percent fat, 0 percent sugar) to 1.0 (0 percent fat, 100 percent sugar). In my clinic, I measured six individuals and compared their fat- and sugar-burning with their primary signs and symptoms, as indicated in the chart below. The pattern of increased fat-burning being coupled with fewer signs and symptoms of fatigue, pain, etc. (i.e., better health) is typical of what I've observed throughout my career.

Signs and symptoms associated with fat- and sugar-burning in six randomly chosen patients:

Patient	Fat-Burning	Sugar-Burning	Signs/Symptoms
JC	12 percent	88 percent	Extreme fatigue, insomnia, 45 pounds overweight.
BK	26 percent	74 percent	Afternoon and evening fatigue, asthma, headaches.
JO	38 percent	62 percent	Afternoon fatigue, allergies, 10 pounds overweight.
PS	45 percent	55 percent	Chronic, mild knee pain, indigestion.
MK	58 percent	42 percent	Occasional low-back pain.
BE	63 percent	37 percent	None.

A KETONE BODY

As we burn higher amounts of body fat, our metabolism significantly increases the production of ketone bodies—a group of three natural chemicals produced in the liver from fats. They are an important source of energy. *Nutritional ketosis* is the healthy, metabolic state associated with the production of a high amount of ketone bodies. It may be an important marker, a sign that you have reached a very high level of fat-burning associated with a very low amount of carbohydrate consumption.

Nutritional ketosis could result in even more energy and health benefits as the heart, liver, intestines, and other areas of the body benefit from ketone bodies. This is particularly important for the brain. Ketosis is associated with increased energy for the brain, and can also help reduce inflammation and oxygen radicals, both known to impair function.

The most popular way to determine whether your body is in a state of nutritional ketosis is through a simple dipstick test. Available in drugstores, this evaluates the presence of ketone bodies in urine. But it is only a general measure, albeit one that is adequate in most cases. To more accurately assess ketone bodies levels, blood tests are most valuable, but usually not required.

The numerous health benefits of ketosis really go hand in hand with the benefits of increased fat-burning and reduced reliance on sugar. In addition to the reduction of excess body fat and preventing the overfat condition, ketosis can help suppress hunger. Nutritional ketosis has also been used to help prevent and treat many of the common chronic diseases from Alzheimer's to cancer, and diabetes to heart disease. Here is a short summary:

- **Blood sugar.** Balancing blood sugar is not only important in those with type 2 diabetes, where patients have
successfully reduced or eliminated the need for insulin
injections, but in preventing it. In addition, early stages
of blood sugar problems are often associated with abnormally low levels, sometimes producing sleepiness or
poor concentration after meals, fatigue between meals,
excessive hunger, and other symptoms that affect quality
of life. (Type 1 diabetics have also greatly benefited from
reducing carbohydrate foods and increasing fat-burning
and ketosis—something a knowledgeable health practitioner can help with.)
- **The brain.** The increased use of ketones and decreased
reliance on glucose for energy in the brain also provides
other recognized benefits referred to as *neuroprotection*.
From Alzheimer's disease and other cognitive dysfunction to Parkinson's, most brain problems are preventable.
Protecting the brain is one way to accomplish this, and
a healthy eating plan promoting high fat-burning and
ketosis can have great therapeutic value. Other brain
and head conditions that have responded well to ketosis
include headache, seizures, traumatic brain injury, sleep
disorders, cancer, autism, and multiple sclerosis. In
addition, better learning and concentration is another
benefit.
- **Cardiovascular disease.** The high fat-burning, nutritional ketosis can quickly and significantly reduce a
variety of cardiovascular risk factors. These include
reductions in triglycerides and LDL and total cholesterol
(with an increase in the "good" HDL cholesterol), and
reduction of abnormally high blood pressure. People
should be cautioned that this sometimes happens in a

few days too, so monitoring blood pressure regularly is important.

- **Cancer.** Sugar consumption is positively associated with cancer in humans, and reducing sugar consumption has been used to successfully prevent and treat various cancers. Tumors are known to rely on sugar for their rapid growth, and the strategy that includes nutritional ketosis is to reduce the available sugar and starve the cancer cells, while providing the body with more than adequate energy from fat and ketones.
- In many individuals, nutritional ketosis can quickly and significantly improve carbohydrate intolerance.

It is not necessary to be in a state of nutritional ketosis to reap the benefits of high fat-burning to reduce excess body fat, although these high levels have successfully been used to treat obesity and various diseases. As you determine the level of carbohydrate intake that's best for you, eliminating junk food and adjusting the intake of natural carbohydrates, ketone bodies will rise, sometimes to a moderate or even high levels, something that's perfectly fine. To emphasize: *the purpose of reducing carbohydrate intake is not necessarily to be in ketosis, although it sometimes occurs, but to determine your best eating plan, and an alternative to blindly following a "diet" not specifically tailored for your particular needs.*

To simplify this discussion, let's just accept that as fat-burning increases there is also a rise in ketone bodies. Nutritional ketosis can be measured, discussed, understood, but be sure not to become obsessed and refer to what you eat as part of a "ketogenic diet." (There are occasionally times when following more precise guidelines are important to assure a high level of ketosis, such as beginning treatment for a seizure disorder, cancer therapy, or others intense therapies. In this situation, a health-care professional can help with the consumption of more measurable amounts of carbohydrates, proteins, and fats to assure the correct outcome is achieved.)

SEVEN SIGNS OF FAT-BURNING

While obtaining a precise measure of how much fat you're burning is ideal, there are clues to when the body starts burning more fat. These come in the form of various signs and symptoms. Here are seven common indications:

1. Clothes fitting more loosely, especially around the waist. While fat doesn't weigh as much as muscle, it can take up more space.
2. People start asking you if you're losing weight. They often notice you are leaner in your face first, and sometimes in other places.
3. Likewise, some people may ask if you're lifting weights; even a slight reduction in body fat can lead to more muscle definition all over.
4. Improved physical and mental performance—increased physical energy leads to less fatigue, and more mental energy, improving brain power, reducing feelings of depression, with overall physical and mental performance boosted.
5. Exercise performance improves. We can walk, run, or bike farther and faster at the same effort or heart rate (discussed later).
6. Increased physical activity without the need for food intake. This might mean longer work periods, travel, or exercise sessions that are more energized with less fatigue.

7. Reduced hunger, which is associated with reduced cravings for sweets.

Of course, a variety of health factors can improve once fat-
burning increases. These can include blood fats (especially triglycerides but cholesterol too), blood pressure, inflammatory-
related conditions, especially pain, intestinal discomfort, sleep
quality, and many others.

BENEFITS OF STORED BODY FAT

It's important to understand that *healthy* body fat serves
many important purposes, until we have too much of it. Here
are some of the health benefits provided by our fat stores:

Insulation. The body's ability to store fat permits humans to live
in most climates, especially in areas of extreme heat or cold. In
warmer areas of the world, stored fat provides protection from
the heat. In colder lands, increased fat stored beneath the skin
prevents too much heat from leaving the body. An example of
fat's effectiveness as an insulator is in the Eskimos' ability to
withstand great cold and survive in good health. Eskimos eat a
high-fat diet, but metabolize (burn) fat well, a reason they have
a low incidence of heart disease and other ailments.

In warmer climates, fat prevents too much water from
leaving the body, which can result in dehydration that causes
dry, scaly skin. Some evaporation is normal, of course, but fats
under the skin regulate evaporation and can prevent as much
as ten to twenty times more water from leaving the body.

The Brain. Over 60 percent of the non-water part of a healthy
brain is fat. During our own development, the incorporation

of fat into the brain enabled us to better create, learn, remember, and grow our brains at a much faster rate. This is especially important for all children from birth, but all adults as well.

The covering of neurons—the specialized brain cells that communicate with each other—have a high fat content, the same type of fat found in olive oil, almonds, and avocados. EPA and DHA, found in fish, are two very common types of fat used by the brain.

Healthy Skin and Hair. Fat has protective qualities that give skin the soft, smooth, and unwrinkled appearance that many people try to achieve through expensive skin conditioners. The healthy look of skin and hair comes from the fat inside our bodies. Fats, particularly cholesterol, serve as an insulating barrier within the skin. Without this protection, chemical pollutants can more easily enter the body through the skin. Hair loss starts with an imbalance of dietary fats that triggers inflammation in the scalp.

Pregnancy and Lactation. The effective functioning of fat-dependent hormones improves fertility for both would-be parents. From conception, fats play a key role in the health of mother and child. The uterus keeps the newly conceived embryo thriving by providing nutrition until the placenta can begin to function, usually a period of a week or more. Adequate progesterone, a hormone produced from fats, is primary for the embryo to survive, preventing miscarriage (spontaneous abortion). Following birth, breastfeeding helps protect the baby against allergies, asthma, and intestinal problems through its high fat content, particularly cholesterol. The baby is highly dependent upon the fat in the milk for survival, especially during the first few days. During this time, the fatty colostrum content of breast milk is of vital nutritional importance.

Body Support and Protection. Stored fat offers physical support and protection to vital body parts, including the organs and glands. Fat acts as a natural, built-in shock absorber, cushioning the wear and tear of everyday life, and helps

---

SICK BODY FAT

Healthy levels of body fat function as an active metabolic system, but excess fat stores can lead to a dysfunction called "adiposopathy," or "sick fat." Without a healthy body, we can also have unhealthy body fat. Excess body fat is the most common cause of poor fat function, which includes diminished fat-burning and a lack of the normal body fat benefits noted above.

Body fat can become dysfunctional if there is an excess accumulation, the reason people who are of normal weight and not obese can be overfat. This is particularly true of excess belly fat.

The excess accumulation of fat can render former healthy fat cells to become literally sick. This results from cellular biochemical alterations leading to adiposopathy. This condition can increase the risk of diabetes, hypertension, high blood cholesterol and triglycerides, and other problems. This can also lead to fat depositing in areas of the body where it does not normally accumulate, causing "lipotoxicity." In addition to more belly fat, other examples include abnormal accumulations of fat in the liver, muscles, pancreas, kidneys, blood vessels, and elsewhere. It can even trigger dysfunction in the associated organs and glands, and further contribute to chronic low-grade inflammation. Sarcopenic obesity is a common condition of aging, a state of combined excess muscle loss and fat accumulation around muscles. It is becoming a more serious problem with increasing levels of chronic disease and an aging population.

---

prevent organs from sinking with age due to the downward pull of gravity.

Fats can physically protect our cells against the harmful effects of X-ray exposure through the control of chemical free-radicals. This includes cosmic radiation from the atmosphere, which penetrates most objects, including airplanes. The average person gets more cosmic radiation exposure during an airline flight from New York to Los Angeles than from a lifetime of medical X-rays.

These and other benefits of stored body fat occur when we have healthy fat cells. Unfortunately, being overfat can impair many of these potential benefits because fat cells become sick.

TWO TYPES OF BODY FAT

The human body possesses two distinct types of body fat, referred to as brown and white. Both are metabolically active, living parts of us.

The attributes of white fat were noted above, in particular the ability to *oxidize* or burn it for energy.

Brown fat makes up only about one percent of the total body fat in healthy adults, with much higher amounts at birth in healthy babies. Brown fat helps us burn white fat. Without brown fat's metabolic action, we can gain body fat and become sluggish in the winter like a hibernating animal. There are a number of ways to increase brown fat activity.

- Eating more frequently—five to six smaller healthy meals instead of one, two, or three larger ones—can trigger *thermogenesis*, an important post-meal metabolic boost to increase fat-burning. However, if caloric intake is too low, brown fat can slow the burning of white fat. This can happen on a low-calorie diet and when meals are skipped.

- The body's brown fat is stimulated by dietary fats, especially those from fish oil and olive oil.
- Caffeine, contained in tea, coffee, and cacao, can increase brown fat activity. But too much caffeine can trigger stress, reducing fat-burning. See sidebar below.
- Refined carbohydrates, including sugar, can quickly reduce fat-burning.

CAN COFFEE IMPROVE FAT-BURNING?

Yes! Caffeine and fat are potent metabolism stimulators.

Properly roasted well-brewed organic coffee is high on my list of life's pleasures. The smell of aromatic beans as I carefully remove them from jar to grinder each morning brings a smile to my face. It continues with the intense taste of the first sip, through the last drop, and beyond. The healthy therapeutic effects on my brain and body still continue to amaze me.

Coffee is among the most studied food in science. One of its well-known abilities is to promote fat-burning. As the beverage highest in caffeine, it has been shown to reduce stored body fat, especially belly fat, and lower the risk of diabetes, liver and colon cancer, cardiovascular disease, and chronic inflammation.

Coffee polyphenols—naturally occurring phytonutrients in the bean—also can help regulate body-wide fat metabolism, improve regulation of insulin and glucose, and help to reduce the tendency toward fat storage and cardiovascular disease as well.

But this does not mean adding sugar to your coffee or making it part of a diet of junk food is going to burn body fat, as refined carbohydrates will easily negate the potential health benefits and in turn ruin a great cup of coffee.

Of course, too much caffeine can be unhealthy for people who are much more sensitive to it than others. It can overstimulate the brain and adrenal glands, revving up the sympathetic nervous system too much and creating an autonomic imbalance. These problems can quickly lead to reduced health. Consuming coffee wisely—drinking the amount that has positive health effects and no more—is part of a healthy diet.

Similar fat-burning and other health benefits have been shown with the various types of caffeinated teas, including black and green. (I like adding a bit of organic raw butter in my tea.)

Clearly coffee can be an amazing fat-burning elixir when used responsibly and combined with healthy fats. Could there be any more pleasurable and tasty component to a healthy diet? Below is my coffee recipe, which I make each morning, and essentially serves as my breakfast. (If you're not eating really well, don't try this at home—or anywhere else!):

Phil's Fat-Burning Organic Coffee
Made from 1½ cups of strong coffee.

In a tall jar or blender, add:
- About ¼ cup heavy cream.
- One raw egg yolk (or very soft-cooked whole egg).
- About one tablespoon of coconut oil.
- About a teaspoon of ground or shaved raw unsweetened cacao.

Add 2–3 tablespoons of hot coffee and blend (I use a hand blender). Add the remaining coffee, pour into a relaxing mug, and enjoy!

Brown fat activity can be easily affected by conscious actions. If we get too hot during the day, or overdress during exercise, brown-fat activity can be reduced. Soaking in a sauna, hot tub, or steam room regularly after exercise may offset some of its fat-burning benefits. Though hot tubs and saunas do come with health benefits, in order to avoid the reductions in fat-burning, take a minute or two to cool the body in a cold shower or tub afterwards.

Conversely, cold stimulates brown fat. Most of our brown fat is found under the skin around the shoulders and underarms, between the ribs, and at the nape of the neck. Cooling these areas can help increase fat-burning. Physical activity increases fat-burning too. The best kind is the easy aerobic type, such as walking.

Burning more body fat for fuel can help increase energy, reduce hunger, and restore normal fat function. The process begins with avoiding junk food. Determining your particular level of carbohydrate intolerance, which is also an important component to the process, is discussed next.

CHAPTER 5

PERSONALIZE YOUR FOOD PLAN WISELY

START WITH THE TWO-WEEK TEST

Once you've taken that first big step—removing refined carbohydrates, including added sugars and other junk food from your life—you most likely will immediately start burning more body fat, storing less, getting leaner, and becoming healthier. It's amazing how many miraculous effects I've seen after this one significant step. It begins a journey of better health and fitness, and causes you to rely on habits such as label-reading and learning to better understand your body and brain, while always being aware that Big Sugar wants to get you back as a customer.

Now you're ready for the second step, determining your level of carbohydrate intolerance, which will help you fine-tune your metabolism even more.

Specifically, this step can help you discover how much *natural* carbohydrate foods such as fruit, lentils, beans, natural grains, honey, and others you tolerate, without even experiencing mild adverse effects. In the early 1980s I developed a process whereby an individual can evaluate themselves—feel what's it's like to be affected by too much carbohydrate. It's called the Two-Week Test.

The Two-Week Test can help you understand your level of carbohydrate intolerance. Discovering whether you are intolerant to a certain amount of natural carbohydrate foods is the next step to further improving fat-burning. Please remember that this is only a test and certainly not a diet, and it will only last two weeks, plus a short follow-up period where you further individualize food choices. It is not the purpose of the Two-Week Test to restrict calories or fat. It merely restricts the many refined carbohydrate junk foods, and even the natural ones. And, there's no need to weigh food or count calories. Just eat what you're allowed, and avoid what's restricted for a period of two weeks. You should not experience hunger during the Two-Week Test—you can eat as much of the non-carbohydrate foods as you want, and as often as you need. If you do become hungry, most likely something isn't just right. This could signal a lack of food intake, especially fats, which reduce hunger, or a sign that you're consuming hidden sugars or other carbohydrates without realizing it.

It's important to understand that the purpose of this test is not to avoid all dietary carbohydrates, or go into nutritional ketosis like with some diet programs whose long-term success is questionable; in fact, once someone goes off one of these diets, weight gain is typical.

Many thousands of people have used my Two-Week Test to get healthy, fit, and significantly improve their energy levels. Others have found it to be the best way to quickly start burning body fat. Still others have reduced or eliminated medications they no longer required. Of all the clinical tools I developed and used for assessment and therapy throughout my career, the consistent results from the Two-Week Test surprised me the most—and still do—specifically regarding how a person can go from one extreme of poor health to vibrant health in such a short time. It's simply a matter of removing a major stress—refined carbohydrates—in a person's life and allowing the body to function the way it was originally meant.

TWO-WEEK TEST GUIDELINES

Before you start the Two-Week Test, plan. First, make a list of any health problems that you might have. This can include symptoms such as fatigue, sleepiness after meals, insomnia, or others from the carbohydrate intolerance survey in chapter 3. In addition, include information if you have specific conditions such as asthma or allergies, migraines, pain, or others. This list may take some time, so don't rush it. This is important because after the Test, you will review these signs and symptoms to see which ones have improved and which have not.

There are two other related items to consider:

- If your blood pressure has been high, and especially if you are on medication, ask your health-care professional to check it soon after starting the test, and especially right after the test. Sometimes high blood pressure normalizes quickly, and your medication may need to be adjusted, or eliminated, which should only be done by your health-care professional. For many people, as insulin levels are reduced to normal, high blood pressure lowers too.

- Hormones become more balanced during the Test, and for women of childbearing age this may mean being more fertile. (The Test has become popular for women who are infertile for the same reason.)

Next, measure your waist circumference before starting the Test. It's something good to do monthly as previously discussed.

As an option, I sometimes recommend writing down your weight before and comparing afterwards—but not during the Test. It's the only instance I recommend using the scale for body weight—but only as a pre- and post-evaluation. During the Test you may lose some excess water your body is holding, which will show on the scale, but you'll also go into a high fat-burning state and start losing body fat. I've seen some people lose only a few pounds during the test, and some twenty or more pounds. *This is not a weight-loss regime, and the main purpose of weighing yourself is to have another sign of how your body is responding after the Test.*

Next, check your food supply. Before you start the test, make sure you have enough of the foods you'll be eating during the test—these are listed below. Go shopping and stock up on these healthy items. Maintain a shopping list of the foods you want to eat and the meals and snacks you want to make available. In addition, go through your cabinets and refrigerator and get rid of junk food: any sweets, foods containing them, and all breads and products made from refined flour. Otherwise, you'll be tempted. Many people are addicted to sugar and other carbohydrates, and for the first few days without them you may crave these foods.

Planning what to eat and how often is important. Schedule the Test during a two-week period that you are relatively unlikely to have distractions—the holidays or times when social engagements are planned can make it too easy to stray from the plan. Don't worry about cholesterol, fat, calories, or the amount of food you're eating. This is only a test, not the way you'll be eating all the time.

Plan to eat at least three meals a day, with some snacks. Most importantly, eat breakfast within an hour of waking, or make the Phil's Fat-Burning Organic Coffee recipe as your breakfast.

Following the Test for less than two weeks probably will not give you a valid result. So, if after five days, for example, you eat a bowl of pasta or a box of cookies, you will need to start the Test over.

FOODS TO EAT DURING THE TEST

You may eat as much of these foods as you like during the Two-Week Test:

- Eggs (whites and yolk), unprocessed (real) cheeses, heavy (whipping) cream, sour cream.
- Unprocessed meats including beef, turkey, chicken, lamb, fish, and shellfish.
- Tomato, V-8, or other vegetable juices except carrot.
- Water—drink it throughout the day in between meals.
- Cooked or raw vegetables such as squash, leaf lettuce and spinach, carrots, broccoli, and kale, but no potatoes or corn.

- Nuts, seeds, nut butters.
- Oils, vinegar, mayonnaise, salsa, mustard, and spices.
- Sea salt, unless you are sodium-sensitive.
- All coffee and tea (if you normally drink it).

Be sure to read the ingredients for all foods, as some form of sugar or carbohydrate may be added. These include peanut butter, mayonnaise, sour cream, and even sliced meats.

FOODS TO AVOID DURING THE TEST

You may *not* eat any of the following foods during the Two-Week Test:

- Bread, rolls, pasta, pancakes, cereal, muffins, chips, crackers, rice cakes, and similar carbohydrate foods
- Sweets such as cake, cookies, ice cream, candy, gum, and breath mints
- Products that contain hidden sugars, common in ketchup and other prepared foods (read the labels)
- Fruits and fruit juice
- Processed meats and fish such as cold cuts and smoked products, which often contain sugar
- All types of potatoes, corn, rice, and beans
- Milk, half-and-half, and yogurt
- So-called healthy snacks, including all energy bars and sports drinks
- All soda; this includes "enhanced" mineral water and diet drinks

A NOTE ON ALCOHOL

If you normally drink small to moderate amounts of alcohol, defined as one drink for women, two for men, some forms are allowed during the test.

> *Alcohol allowed*: dry wines, pure distilled spirits (gin, vodka, whiskey, etc.), and those mixed with plain carbonated water, including seltzer, tomato juice, or V-8.

> *Alcohol not allowed:* Sweet wines, all beer, champagne, alcohol containing sugar, including all liqueurs, and those mixed with sweet ingredients such as tonic, soda, or other sugary liquids. If in doubt, avoid it.

Below are some other suggestions for eating, food preparation, and dining out that may be helpful during the Two-Week Test. You may find these suggestions useful after completing the test as well.

MEAL IDEAS

Eggs
- Omelets, with any combination of vegetables, meats, and cheeses
- Scrambled with guacamole, sour cream, and salsa
- Scrambled with a scoop of ricotta cheese and tomato sauce
- Boiled or poached with spinach or asparagus and hollandaise or cheese sauce; with bacon or other meats
- Soufflés

Salads
- Chef—leaf lettuce, meats, cheeses, eggs
- Spinach—with bacon, eggs, anchovies
- Caesar—Romaine lettuce, eggs, Parmesan cheese, anchovies
- Any salad with chicken, tuna, shrimp, or other meat or cheese

Salad Dressings
- Extra-virgin olive oil and vinegar (balsamic, wine, apple cider). Plain or with sea salt and spices
- Creamy—made with heavy cream, mayonnaise, garlic, and spices

Fish and Meats
- Pot roast cooked with onions, carrots, and celery
- Roasted chicken stuffed with a bulb of anise, celery, and carrots
- Chili-type dish made with fresh, chopped meat and a variety of vegetables such as diced eggplant, onions, celery, peppers, zucchini, tomatoes, and spices (no beans)
- Steak and eggs
- Any meat with a vegetable and a mixed salad
- Chicken parmigiana (not breaded or deep-fried) with a mixed salad
- Fish (not breaded or deep-fried) with any variety of sauces and vegetables
- Tuna melt on a bed of broccoli or asparagus

Sauces
- Plain melted butter
- A quick cream sauce can be made by simmering heavy cream with mustard or curry powder and cayenne

pepper, or any flavor of choice. It's delicious over eggs, poultry, and vegetables
- Italian-style tomato sauce helps makes a quick parmigiana out of any fish, meat, or vegetables. Put this over spaghetti squash for a pasta-like dish. Or make lasagna with sliced grilled eggplant or zucchini instead of pasta

Snacks
- Hard-boiled eggs
- Rolled slices of fresh meat and/or cheese wrapped in lettuce
- Vegetable juices
- Raw almonds, cashews, pecans
- Celery stuffed with nut butter or cream cheese
- Guacamole with vegetable sticks for dipping
- Leftovers from a previous meal

Dining Out
- Let the waiter know you do not want any bread or bread sticks, to avoid temptation
- Ask for an extra vegetable instead of rice or potato
- Chinese: Steamed meat, fish, or vegetables (no rice or sweet sauce)
- Continental: steak, roast, duck, fish, or seafood
- French: coquille Saint Jacques, beef Bourguignonne
- Italian: Veal parmigiana (not breaded or deep-fried), seafood marinara
- Beware that most tomato sauces have added sugar

Avoid all fried food, as it usually has breading or is coated in flour.

AFTER THE TEST

Following the Two-Week Test, reevaluate your original list of signs and symptoms. Is your energy level better? Are you sleeping better? Feeling less depressed? If you feel better now than you did two weeks ago, or if you lost weight, you probably have a moderate degree of carbohydrate intolerance and you're unable to eat as many carbohydrates as you did before the test. Some people who have a high degree of CI will feel dramatically better than they did before the Test, especially if there was a large weight loss. Some people say they feel like a new person after taking this Test. Others say after a few days of the Test they feel young again.

Any weight loss during the Test is not due to reduced calories, as many people eat more calories than usual during this two-week period. It's due to the increased fat-burning resulting from reduced insulin. While there may be some water loss, especially if you are sodium sensitive, there is *real* fat loss.

If nothing improved during the test—and it was done exactly as described above—then you may not be very carbohydrate intolerant. It may be that the level of natural carbohydrates you are consuming, and considering that you no longer eat junk food, is appropriate for your needs.

But if the Two-Week Test improved at least some of your signs and symptoms, the next step is to determine how much carbohydrate your body can tolerate, without a return of the original signs and symptoms that have now improved or disappeared.

At this stage, having just completed the test, your body and brain will be more aware of even slight reactions to carbohydrate foods. Basically, your instincts will be more active and you'll be more aware to how your body responds to food. This step is done in the following manner over the next one to two weeks:

- Begin adding single-serving amounts of natural, unprocessed carbohydrates at every other meal or snack. This may be plain yogurt sweetened with a little honey for breakfast, or an apple after lunch or dinner
- For a snack, try tea with honey or fruit
- Avoid all refined carbohydrates such as sugar and refined-flour products (like white bread, cereals, rolls, or pasta)
- Other suggestions include brown rice, sweet potatoes, yams, lentils, and beans

Most bread, crackers, cereals, and other grains are processed and should be avoided—even those stating "whole grain" or "100 percent whole wheat." Read the ingredients carefully. If you can find real-food whole grain products, they can be used. These include sprouted breads, whole oats (they take about 45 minutes to cook), and other dense products made with just ground wheat, rye, or other grains. If in doubt, avoid them during this one- to two-week period.

I want to emphasize again not to add carbohydrates in back-to-back meals or snacks because insulin production is partly influenced by your previous meal.

With the addition of natural carbohydrates, be aware of any symptoms you had previously that were eliminated by the test, especially symptoms that develop immediately after eating, such as intestinal bloating, sleepiness, or feelings of depression.

Most importantly, if any signs or symptoms that disappeared during or following the Two-Week Test have now returned during this follow-up period, you've probably exceeded your carbohydrate limit. For example, if your hunger or cravings were mostly eliminated at the end of the Two-Week Test, and now they've returned, you probably added too many carbohydrates. If you lost eight pounds during the test, and gained back five pounds after adding some carbohydrates for a week or two, you've probably eaten too many of them. Likewise, if blood pressure rises significantly after it was reduced, it may be due to excess carbohydrate intake. If any of these situations occur, reduce the carbohydrates by half, or otherwise, experiment to see which particular foods cause symptoms and which don't. Some people return to the Two-Week Test and begin the process again.

In some cases, people can tolerate simple carbohydrates, such as fresh fruits or honey, but not complex carbohydrates such as sweet potato, whole grains, beans, or other starches. This may be due to the difficulty in digesting starches in some people with CI. In other situations, some individuals can't tolerate any wheat products due to a sensitivity or even allergy to gluten. During this post-test period, these dietary factors are usually easy to determine.

After a one- to two-week period following the Two-Week Test, by experimenting with natural carbohydrates you'll have a much better idea about your body's level of tolerance. You'll better know which foods to avoid, which ones you can eat, and those that must be limited. You'll become acutely aware of how your body feels when you eat too many carbohydrates.

From time to time, you may feel the need to go through a Two-Week Test period again to check yourself, or to quickly get back on track after careless eating such as during the holidays, vacations, or periods of stress.

GUT FUNCTION

Many people find the loss of grains in the diet leaves the digestive tract sluggish and a little constipated. While this is often something that corrects itself, after years of eating lots of carbohydrates, your intestine gets used to that type of food. If you become constipated during the Two-Week Test, or afterwards when a lower amount of carbohydrate in the diet is maintained, it could be due to a number of reasons:

- First, you may not be eating enough fiber. Bread, pasta, and cereals are significant sources of fiber.
- You may not be eating enough of other foods that improve gut function, especially fat and vegetables.
- Dehydration may be another reason for constipation at this time. If you don't drink enough water, you could be predisposed to constipation.
- Psyllium is a high-fiber herb that is an effective promoter of intestinal function. Adding plain unsweetened psyllium to a glass of water, tomato juice, or healthy smoothie can keep your system running smoothly. Start with a half teaspoon a day for a few days to make sure it's tolerated, then slowly increase and use up to a couple of teaspoons (only occasionally do people respond best with up to one tablespoon a day). Another way to add psyllium to your diet is to use it in place of flour for thickening sauces or in place of bread crumbs to coat meats and vegetables. If you require a fiber supplement, be sure to use the ones that do not contain sugar, so read the labels.

Occasionally, some people get tired during or after the Two-Week Test. Most commonly it's from not eating enough food, and/or not eating often enough. The most common problem is not eating breakfast. Also, many people should not go more than three to four hours without eating something healthy.

MAINTAINING CARBOHYDRATE BALANCE

Once you successfully finish the Two-Week Test and add back the right amount of tolerable carbohydrate foods, you should have an excellent idea of your carbohydrate limits— the amount of carbohydrate you can eat without producing abnormal signs or symptoms. This is best accomplished by consistently assessing your levels of mental and physical energy, sleepiness, and bloating after meals, or any of the problems you had previous to taking the Two-Week Test. Initially, you may want to keep a diary so you can be more objective in your self-assessment. In time, you won't need to focus as much on this issue as your intuition will take over and you'll automatically know your limits.

Once you find your level of carbohydrate tolerance, you're on your way to balancing your whole diet. Yet another important aspect of carbohydrate foods to be more aware of is which of the many choices available in supermarkets, farmer's markets, and elsewhere are truly healthy, and which to avoid. While there's nothing radical about the notion that refined carbohydrates are unhealthy, there are many radical diet plans that make it seem like all carbohydrates are deadly. They're not. Finding your level of tolerance is what's most important, then eat only healthy carbohydrates.

To summarize, here are the basics of the Two-Week Test:
- Write a list of all your signs and symptoms
- Measure your waist and weigh yourself
- Plan your meals and snacks—buy sufficient foods allowed on the test, and get rid of those not allowed so you're not tempted
- Eat as much as you need, and as often as you need, to never get hungry

WHAT IS LOW-CARB?

Many low-carbohydrate diets have come and gone for decades, only with different names—low-carb, caveman, ketogenic, and others. They are nothing new. The fact is, low-carb eating is how humans ate for millions of years. While modern diets may have had short-term success rates, they were not healthy because they didn't teach us about healthy eating; most of these diets include a lot of unhealthy processed foods. In addition, this approach usually doesn't address sugar addiction. Plus, they tended to be deficient in essential fats and other nutrients.

As emphasized throughout this book, self-health management allows you to return to nature, follow instincts and intuition, and eat the way your body wants based on healthy needs.

To put this approach into perspective, I offer some common definitions. You may hear some of these terms, although they often appear without clear definitions. They will help you on your journey to burn more body fat and get lean and healthy.

- Low-carb: About 11–25 percent of daily meals, with approximately 51–139 grams of natural carbohydrates per day. This would bring fat content to between 135 and 165 grams, or about 58–71 percent.
- Very low-carb: about 5–10 percent of daily meals, with around 25–50 grams of natural carbohydrates. Fats are about 168–182 grams, about 72–78 percent. At this level of carbohydrate intake, we make many more ketone bodies for energy for use by the heart, liver, brain, and other tissues.

Very low-carb also refers to:

- Ketogenic eating—a state of healthy nutritional ketosis.
- High-fat—Obviously, if carbohydrates are reduced to 25 percent or less of the diet, with protein holding steady, the fat content will increase to higher levels. With "normal" fat intake considered to be 30 percent, low-fat is below that level with high-fat well above. Don't be concerned about eating this much natural, healthy fat.

- Always eat breakfast
- After the test, reevaluate your signs and symptoms, including weight
- Begin adding natural, unprocessed carbohydrates to every other meal or snack, and evaluate whether this causes any of your previous signs or symptoms (or weight) to return

The Two-Week Test was primarily developed for adults, despite the fact that millions of children are overfat. Eliminating junk food is often enough to significantly improve the lives of children, and correct or prevent the overfat condition.

CHAPTER 6

OVERFAT CHILDREN

Virtually all health organizations, clinicians, and scientists, not to mention many parents, know that the rise in the prevalence of overweight and obese children, and the even higher levels of overfat children who have related diseases, is past the point of being serious. It's one of the most alarming public health issues facing the world today. And it's what is feeding the overfat pandemic. What's even worse is that overfat children are now developing adult diseases and, unfortunately, most of these overfat children remain that way into adulthood.

In the US, over 30 percent of children are overweight or obese, with much larger numbers—over 50 percent—being overfat. While this is a terrifying figure, only more recently has the problem taken on a new twist.

As a result of being overfat, increasing numbers of children are developing conditions that used to be only found in adults.

Type 2 diabetes *used* to be referred to as adult-onset diabetes. But no more, as this and other diseases are showing up in children.

Along with type 2 diabetes, children are being diagnosed with conditions such as high blood pressure, high cholesterol and triglycerides, sleep apnea, and other conditions, all more typically associated with adults. Many of these are a part of the metabolic syndrome.

A recent report by the nonprofit *Fair Health*, a national clearinghouse for health claims data, showed that claims for type 2 diabetes among people 22 years old and younger more than doubled between 2011 and 2015.

At the same time, claims for pre-diabetes among children rose 110 percent, while high blood pressure claims rose 67 percent. Sleep apnea, an associated condition in which a patient temporarily stops breathing while sleeping, rose 161 percent.

The analysis also found that during the four years analyzed, the number of claims tied to obesity diagnosis jumped 94 percent among infants and toddlers.

Virtually all these conditions are found in those who are carbohydrate intolerant and overfat.

The results are even more frightening, as these children may be living shorter lives with a lower quality of life.

There's good news: as easy as it is to make changes in adults, it can be even easier in children.

HEALTHIER CHILDREN IN TEN DAYS

Like the Two-Week Test in adults, who can become significantly better in that short time frame, children can sometimes do even better.

A recent study published in the journal *Obesity* showed that overfat children who stopped eating added sugars for just ten days dramatically improved their health. It wasn't just an "improvement," and the word "dramatic" does not do the results justice. The majority of those children in the study group actually reversed chronic cardiac and metabolic disease indicators, such as high levels of cholesterol, high blood pressure, high blood sugar and insulin, liver dysfunction, and other problems in just ten days.

Metabolic syndrome comprises a cluster of disease risk factors including hypertension, altered glucose metabolism, high blood fats, increased abdominal fat, and others. It is common in adults but now occurs in children too. What's most remarkable about the children with metabolic syndrome is how quickly they are now developing it.

As dramatic as this study may sound, it's not really new to many clinicians and parents who have already experienced this phenomenon. But for many people who read the headlines, this may come as an almost unbelievable shock—one simple dietary change and a ten-day duration make this big of a difference? It's almost too good to be true.

While I've observed similar changes in adults, it should also not be surprising that sugar and flour, which quickly turns to sugar when eaten, is that bad for the body. It's why the white stuff has been compared to heroin and cocaine.

My first thought after reading this study was this: Imagine if these kids stopped eating all refined carbohydrates?

Left unchecked, the devastating effects of sugar consumption can lead to pediatric metabolic syndrome, a condition that is also increasing, meaning more children are getting more sick earlier in life. While it's easy to see the problem in an obese child, the lean ones can be affected too, sometimes just as badly. That's because they are overfat.

Metabolic dysfunction early in life can lead to a long list of possible secondary chronic health conditions in adulthood, if not before, including heart disease, diabetes, chronic inflammation, oxidative stress, hypertension, infertility, non-alcoholic fatty liver disease, sleep apnea, Alzheimer's, cancer, and numerous others. These are preventable conditions, and the sooner we begin to address the problems, the easier we can prevent disease.

CATCHING CI EARLY

Long before some children become clearly overfat, many develop various signs and symptoms that make it clear they are at high risk for it. Don't be fooled by those children who are not obese, or who seem to pass their pediatric checkups. Metabolic dysfunctions may be brewing in these young bodies as well. Fortunately, there are clues that there are problems, that carbohydrate intolerance exists.

Like many adults, children can have various signs and symptoms associated with carbohydrate intolerance. These may include excess insulin production (hyperinsulinemia), blood-sugar irregularities, abdominal obesity, and others. Earlier in life there may be other, more objective indicators. They may also have seemingly unrelated conditions, or vague symptoms.

Below is a valuable health survey that lists some of the important clues, in the form of signs and symptoms, in children that may indicate a higher risk of carbohydrate intolerance.

Check the items that apply:

Birth weight: 5½ pounds or less; 9 pounds or more.
Taller than average for age.
Increased body weight or fat.
Parent, grandparent, or sibling is diabetic.
Sleep problems.
Increased aggression or anger.
Brain injury (including learning, behavior, and other
    problems).
Overeating sweets or carbohydrates causes upset.
Physical activity less than 4 hours per week.
Family or personal history of high blood pressure, high
    cholesterol or triglycerides, heart disease, stroke, or
    cancer.
Sweet tooth or sugar-addicted.
Mother: high-stress during pregnancy.

Children with more than two checked items may be at increased risk for carbohydrate intolerance.

Sometimes just one or two of the items in this survey could mean there's an increased risk for carbohydrate intolerance, and certainly the risk may increase with more signs or symptoms. However, just eliminating junk food could make dramatic health changes. How much should you reduce them? The less bad food in the diet the better.

The Two-Week Test, discussed in the last chapter, was designed primarily for adults. Parents who perform this test often realize the health of their children is also being compromised by the intake of too much junk food and make adjustments to their kids' diets as well.

I don't recommend the Two-Week Test for children, although some adolescents might find it useful. The important thing is that children should not eat unhealthy food, and since parents directly influence their eating habits, it's our responsibility to offer healthy foods to our kids. Many of us have children, grandchildren, friends, and family who have children. We all have such a great opportunity to influence them in a significant way.

The foods children eat not only affect their health, but impact their fitness ability too. This generation of children moves slower than their parents.

SLOW CHILDREN AHEAD

We've been seeing the signs for years, that many children are not only overfat, but slower too.

Physical activity levels in children have gradually declined during the decades of the building overfat epidemic. For example, only about half of American children achieve at least sixty minutes of moderate-intensity physical activity daily. Starting in elementary school, activity levels continuously decline. This is, of course, a problem, but the report card gets worse.

What has dramatically changed is *fitness*. The American Heart Association has shown that many children can't run as far or fast as their parents did. In fact, in a one-mile run, today's children are about a minute and a half slower than their peers thirty years ago with average changes similar between boys and girls, younger and older kids.

There's no question that regular physical activity promotes growth and development, with many physical, mental, and psychosocial benefits. It can also contribute to better learning and can reduce the risk for heart disease, diabetes, osteoporosis, high blood pressure, along with metabolic syndrome and the overfat condition. It improves aerobic capacity, muscle and bone strength, flexibility, and can help reduce stress, anxiety, and depression.

All these serious problems in children may reflect increased carbohydrate intake, which reduces fat-burning even more than decreased levels of physical activity. But there's no reason to debate which came first. Children need to eat real food *and* be physically active.

To end the overfat pandemic, we have to stop what's feeding it: overfat children. Helping them get healthy and lean is relatively simple; follow the same plan discussed in this book, although, in many ways it's easier. Since children learn from adults, we have to teach by example. If we eat in a disordered fashion, our children could too.

CHAPTER 7

DISORDERED EATING AND OVERFAT

There's no question that the overfat pandemic is associated with unhealthy eating habits, as discussed earlier in this book. By definition, the consumption of pathogenic food is pathogenic eating, also described as disordered eating.

Mention "eating disorders," and most people think of the serious mental health conditions of anorexia nervosa and bulimia. But milder forms of the condition are more common. Disordered eating appears to be a widespread but well-hidden problem in adolescents and adults, and in both males and females.

As described in the *Diagnostic and Statistical Manual of Mental Disorders* (DSM), eating disorders are characterized by gross disturbances in eating behavior. They include anorexia nervosa, bulimia nervosa, and eating-related problems termed "not otherwise specified."

The American Psychiatric Association says that the "not otherwise specified" category is for eating problems that do not meet all the criteria for any specific eating disorder. These cases, which may make up the majority, are referred to as *subclinical* eating disorders, and sometimes referred to as stress-induced eating. While this category greatly expands the condition of disordered eating to include many more people, perhaps rightly so, it may still not be enough. The problem can be classified in a much simpler way—disordered eating.

Disordered eating is not a single condition but a wide spectrum of maladaptive eating associated with sugar addiction, weight control activity, the use of diets and other unhealthy eating patterns, and misinformation. Just where a person exists on this spectrum, if at all, is often but not always easy to discern. Too many people with disordered eating fall through the cracks of the health-care system. Of course, our society, whether directly or indirectly, even encourages disordered eating. Big Sugar promotes it, and has lobbied governments to twist dietary recommendation in their favor.

For many people with disordered eating, they don't recognize the problem as unhealthy. Only when a full-blown clinical diagnosis is made does it become obvious.

Eating disorders are sometimes referred to as pathogenic eating because the outcome can be poor health and disease. Just a single meal or snack containing refined carbohydrates, especially sugar, can have a measurable pathogenic effect on the body, even in healthy people. In chapter 3, I mentioned that, because junk food is clearly harmful, some health authorities want to call it *pathogenic food*. It makes sense that one who regularly consumes pathogenic food would have pathogenic eating. Let's keep it simple and just call it disordered eating.

Disordered eating includes the consumption of unhealthy food, and can include dieting, calorie restriction, reducing fat intake, fasting (not for health reasons), and the use of laxatives, diuretics, diet pills, and vomiting.

The onset of disordered eating can be during adolescence, particularly in children desiring thinness, weight loss, or for sports-related reasons. It involves being obsessed with avoiding fat calories, dieting, or other unhealthy habits, often influenced by peers or parents.

Many people develop disordered eating as a result of misinformation. Marketing hype and governmental recommendations that evolved from lobbying efforts by Big Sugar may cause most of this distorted information as it pertains to low-fat, low-calorie, and being on a diet. Usually without malice, misinformation can also come from friends and family, or athletes and coaches.

In some cases, disordered eating is an ongoing problem, a regular routine, while at other times it emerges periodically: in the spring to prepare for the summer bathing-suit season, before a big formal event like a wedding or graduation, or, as in the case of athletes, leading up to their competitive seasons. Regardless of the details, the condition creates ill health, especially poor metabolism that impairs fat-burning. This is the reason most people following diets ultimately gain any weight that was lost back again, plus more.

Whether people are aware of it or not, disordered eating is a frustrating condition. It usually does not result in any true success, but often leads to excess stress or even depression, conditions people are more easily aware of.

IS ORTHOREXIA REAL?

While almost all disordered eating is associated with various food *quantity* issues—especially the amounts of calories or fat—a recent name has surfaced that is associated with food *quality*. In clinical terms, *orthorexia nervosa* refers to people who are obsessed with eating healthy food with an unhealthy outcome. However, the term is often improperly used in a more general way on blogs and social media, and even in newspapers and magazines, being applied to anyone who carefully chooses to eat only healthy food. Nevertheless, this is not disordered eating.

Orthorexia nervosa, from the Greek, is translated to mean *correct appetite*. The term may have first appeared in a 1997 article in a yoga magazine as a quote from Dr. Steven Bratman.

Orthorexia is not an official diagnosis in the *Diagnostic and Statistical Manual of Mental Disorders*, and not recognized as an eating disorder by the American Psychiatric Association. The term is starting to appear in published scientific journals but without consensus of its meaning. The prevailing discussions by clinicians and scientists is that orthorexia nervosa is an eating disorder associated with fanatical behavior regarding food quality, and a true obsession leading to an unhealthy outcome. However, in this context, it has not been applied to those who are self-conscious, cautious, and careful to avoid pathogenic eating.

So when and if the term is accepted into scientific circles, it will be used to describe a form of disordered eating that includes abnormal behavior that is potentially harmful, but not applicable to those people with a passion for choosing healthy food over pathogenic food.

A disorder means there's some physical, biochemical, or mental-emotional problem, typically a combination. Depending on the seriousness of the disorder, correcting it may be accomplished by the individual through natural means or with the help of a health-care professional. The first step, of course, is for the individual to understand that there is a genuine problem, and he or she has the desire to remedy it.

TWO FORMS OF DISORDERED EATING

The spectrum of disordered eating is wide, going from mild, almost unnoticeable problems—subclinical disordered eating—to the serious, more recognized clinical conditions.

Subclinical Disordered Eating

As noted above, those with eating and food problems who don't neatly fit into the criteria for named conditions are classified as having a subclinical eating disorder. This condition may exist early in life—during adolescence or even younger—with at least three possible outcomes: 1) the problem precedes a more serious, well-defined clinical mental illness; 2) the condition remains a less-defined subclinical problem; or 3) the problem is resolved.

For those people with a subclinical eating disorder, it may not be recognized as a problem. While many unhealthy attitudes about food may be considered "normal" for athletes or those on a diet, some experts still consider this condition to be a risk factor for more serious clinical eating disorders.

Clinical Disordered Eating

The diagnostic criteria for the two most common clinical disorders are extensive, but here is a review:

- For anorexia nervosa, the criteria include a refusal to maintain body weight at healthy levels, an abnormal fear of gaining weight or body fat, a disturbed image of one's body, and the denial of the seriousness of one's condition. In females this may also include amenorrhea (the absence of menstrual bleeding) or oligomenorrhea (a menstrual cycle between 35 and 90 days), and in younger adolescents, delayed menarche (onset of first period). These patients are classified into the food-restricting type or the binge-eating/purging type.
- The criteria for the diagnosis of bulimia nervosa include recurrent episodes of binge eating (quickly eating large amounts of food) followed by vomiting (purging), which leads to more binge eating. The classification includes the purging and non-purging type.

SUGAR ADDICTION

The few remaining people in the world who have trouble accepting the notion that sugar is so addicting may be in denial. It's not perceived in the same way as tobacco or alcohol. In fact, "more scientific studies are needed to study if sugar is indeed addicting" is the argument often voiced by the sugar industry and its well-paid lobbyists who also exert influence in the media and government. (To this day, the tobacco industry continues to argue that "more studies are needed" to determine whether cigarette smoking or second-hand smoke is truly harmful.)

What is it about sugar that makes it so difficult for many people to wean themselves off it or go "cold turkey"? Does the dependency have to do with a person's sweet tooth? Is the addiction to sweets an acquired habit? And why are some individuals able to live quite happily without sweets as part of their regular diet?

Through the years, I have observed that many people were initially unable to even consider giving up sugar and other refined carbohydrates. Just the thought was much too difficult to contemplate. Even the lure and promise of optimal health, including increased fat-burning, reduced body fat, weight loss, more energy, and better mental focus, was insufficient. They rather remained in the rut of their own choosing.

Many people with a sugar dependency argue that foods don't taste the same without being sweetened. Since sugar is such a widely used ingredient found in many processed products, from so-called "healthy breads" to cereals (even added to "bland" brands like Wheaties and Cheerios) and energy bars to even staples like tomato sauce, finding out which foods don't contain sugar or high-fructose corn syrup is often a challenge.

Scientific research of sugar's chemical effect on the body has shown that it triggers the brain's pleasure and reward centers—emotional areas responsible for the release of a "feel good" neurotransmitter called dopamine. These are the same brain areas stimulated by cocaine, nicotine, opiates (such as heroin and morphine), and alcohol. This addiction is not an imaginary thought in the minds of millions of sugar junkies— it's associated with real physiological changes in the brain. Since the brain's pleasure areas are also close to the pain centers, withdrawal from sugar is often described by many people as being painful—not unlike experiencing romantic pain, the loss of a loved one, or eliminating nicotine or caffeine.

Psychoactive compounds present in cocoa and chocolate, salsolinol being the main one, might be why chocolate can also be so addicting. But the high levels of added sugar contained in most chocolate products are what is probably much more addictive than the chocolate alone. Those who break free of sugar can still enjoy natural cacao, which is the real thing with the tastiest chocolate flavor and health benefits.

Sugar may also be a primary addiction, while others are secondary. In this case, treating the sugar problem might be the first step in eliminating other harmful substances such as alcohol, nicotine, caffeine, or harder drugs like heroin and cocaine. Other modalities such as hypnosis, acupuncture, behavior modification, and psychotherapy can be useful. In my clinical experience, when helping patients who were addicted to drugs—from alcohol to amphetamines and caffeine to cocaine—the most successful cases with a long-term positive outcome were initiated by first eliminating sugar and other refined carbohydrates.

If you are sugar-dependent, ask yourself this: after a big meal of pasta, bread, soft drink, and dessert, does your behavior change? Do you become sleepy, moody, or have a loss of concentration? When you avoid sugar altogether, do you experience cravings? Do you tend to eat sugary foods even though you know you shouldn't, and feel you should better control yourself? Are sweets a comfort food for you? These questions about sugar addiction are similar to indications of drug addiction, and the reason researchers and clinicians see an overlap between sweets and drugs. The sugar-bingeing cycle is perpetuated when sugar is unavailable, which is then followed by the urge to abuse the drug (sugar) again.

Let's look at some behavioral aspects of sugar addiction. Which of these statements applies to you when it comes to eating sugar-containing foods and other refined carbohydrates?

1. Eating until feeling uncomfortably full.
2. Eating large amounts when not physically hungry.
3. Eating much more rapidly than normal.
4. Often eating alone because you're embarrassed by how much you're consuming.
5. Feeling guilty, depressed, or disgusted after overeating.
6. Marked distress or anxiety regarding binge eating.

Binge-eating episodes are associated with three or more of these factors. These questions might provide criteria for a clinical diagnosis of binge-eating with sugar. The most recent edition of the DSM defines binge-eating as a series of recurrent binge episodes in which each one is defined as eating a larger amount of food than normal during any two-hour period. Without any exaggeration, I've been told this identical eating history by thousands of patients throughout my career—people who were not, in my opinion, mentally ill, but were binge-eaters—and for the most part, because they simply couldn't wean themselves from sugar. And people addicted to sugar tend to binge more frequently.

Big Sugar knows sugar is addictive. It's why they make it so readily available, and carefully place sugar-laden foods in easy-to-access locations, such as at the checkout counter, and at eye-level for children to see while sitting in the shopping cart. Those of us who have kicked the habit, and those who have tried many times, also know how addicting it can be. My preferred recommendation, one that clearly has been most effective during my career, is to kick the sugar habit right now. The "cold turkey" approach of just stopping works best, especially when one has a well thought out, organized approach, such as the Two-Week Test.

The concept of managing our own health comes into play with sugar addiction as much as any other aspect of health. The bottom line: it's up to each of us to kick the habit.

DISORDERED EATING AND EXERCISE

Disordered eating is common among people who exercise, including competitive athletes, with estimates by the National Athletic Trainers' Association's position statement that range as high as 62 percent among female and 33 percent among male athletes.

Disordered eating is disordered behavior, and the problem typically reaches beyond one's diet. For example, the overtraining syndrome in both men and women is commonly associated with disordered eating. Unhealthy outcomes, such as amenorrhea, fatigue, physical injury, depression, and others, are typically part of the clinical picture. The need for a holistic approach is essential so all physical, biochemical, and mental-emotional aspects of the individual are addressed.

Exercise is often used as an excuse to eat junk food. Many patients told me that when eating too much sugar, they just make sure they exercise more to "burn off the calories." As discussed in the next chapter, this notion is completely false.

DISORDERED EATING AND LIFESTYLE

An important component of disordered eating is its relationship to behavioral lifestyle disorders. Beyond food, various other aspects of health and fitness may be part of the problem, especially those desiring extreme weight loss and thinness, and increased exercise performance.

Whether cause or effect, three important factors associated with disordered eating include:

- **Sugar addiction.** It would appear that most people with disordered eating have sugar addiction. Many mistakenly believe that only fatty foods add weight and body fat, but can't consider that up to half the refined carbohydrates eaten, those most consumed by people with disordered eating, quickly convert to stored body fat.
- **Stress can also be a significant factor associated with disordered eating.** "Stress may indirectly contribute to disease (e.g., cardiovascular disease, cancer) by producing deleterious changes to diet" (O'Connor, 2015). Human studies have demonstrated increased preference for high-sugar foods in people reporting greater stress exposure, with daily stressors associated with unhealthy snack consumption. Much of this disordered eating is

linked with a negative reward pattern of behavior—the connection with sugar addiction. Of course, most people already know this, and it's an important part of making healthy changes. More importantly, unhealthy eating patterns even result in an increased level of stress, which maintains a vicious cycle not easy to break.

- **Anxiety disorders, mood disorders, and insomnia.** These three problems are mentioned in studies and tend to increase with eating disorders. They are often the end-result of poor brain and body health.

WHAT TO DO?

What may often elude most people with eating disorders is the fact that there is a general consensus among most nutritional scientists and clinicians about healthy eating. This includes avoiding junk food, and the need to regularly consume fresh fruits and vegetables and foods with quality protein and fat, while obtaining at least adequate calories and micronutrients for one's particular needs. So one can be normal weight and lean, and improve exercise performance by eating healthy foods. This understanding is a foundation of natural therapy essential for an individual to avoid disordered eating.

While I don't want to oversimplify a remedy for disordered eating, here are three important starting points for many individuals:

- Recognize the full context of the problem: understand it better.
- Decide to make healthy changes. This recommendation appears straightforward for most with subclinical disorders, but it is not always easy.

- Address the primary issues related to disordered eating, including sugar addiction.

Interestingly, by learning about healthy eating and giving up junk food, you can address sugar addiction and experience improvements in overall health that can often allow the brain and body to function better with the real result of eliminating disordered eating as well. It's perfectly fine and heathy to be passionate about getting and maintaining great health. It's a key part of the journey to reduce excess body fat.

CHAPTER 8

START YOUR FAT-BURNING ENGINES!

The overfat pandemic has not spared those who exercise.

In a society strongly emphasizing health, well-being, and physical performance, it is an unfortunate contradiction that illness, injury, disease, and the overfat pandemic are now the norm.

While eating healthy food can immediately and powerfully stimulate metabolism to burn the right mix of fat and sugar, physical activity can complement it. In fact, fat is burned in muscles, in a complex biochemical process called beta-oxidation. We can influence how much fat and sugar we burn by choosing the appropriate level of intensity during exercise.

Food, however, is still the primary regulator of this process, so even if we perform the perfect exercise but consume refined carbohydrates, especially right before working out, the potential fat-burning benefits of the workout may be reduced. But by avoiding sugar, the right exercise can further enhance the fat-burning process, along with providing other health and fitness benefits.

Fat-burning takes place in the *aerobic* muscle fibers throughout the body. This is called the aerobic engine or system. Burning fat calories is easy—best accomplished during slower, lower intensity activities. Aerobic muscles, also called slow-twitch, are fatigue-resistant; unlike power muscles, they allow us to perform at relatively slow paces all day long.

So say goodbye to no-pain, no-gain high-intensity anaerobic exercise, which means high sugar-burning and less fat-burning. When it comes to working out, don't just do it, do it right!

This means building the aerobic system during periods of low-intensity training and natural movement to improve aerobic function, fat-burning, and health before embarking on higher-intensity activities if that is your desire. Low-intensity workouts might include walking, easy jogging or cycling, swimming, dancing, and others associated with low heart rates. High-intensity means high heart rates usually associated with faster running, cycling, and other activities. (As discussed later, you can still develop speed and power if that's your goal.)

Easy does it: exercise intensity and fat-burning

Intensity	Type	Fuel/calorie mix
Lower	Aerobic	Higher fat-burning/lower sugar-burning
Higher	Anaerobic	Higher sugar-burning/lower fat-burning

Humans are among the most amazing endurance animals on earth. One reason is our built-in ability to have almost unlimited energy for nearly fatigue-free long-term physical activity. This comes from our capacity to use stored body fat for fueling our movements. Even the leanest among us has sufficient body fat to travel on foot for many hundreds of miles.

The aerobic system also helps to stabilize blood sugar, reduce hunger, balance hormones, prevent injuries, improve immune function, and ensure better brain function. Fully developing and properly feeding the aerobic system leads to optimal human performance on all levels.

In addition to eating junk food, another problem has to do with physical activity levels, as represented by two different groups of the population: those who are inactive, and those performing too much high-intensity workout following a no-pain, no-gain approach. In both situations, body fat can accumulate because the fat-burning mechanism does not develop. When this happens, *aerobic deficiency* follows—a problem that almost all overfat people experience.

THE NEW AEROBIC REVOLUTION

Most people think they know what aerobic means (or so they say). Many associate it with breathing or oxygen and confuse it with "cardio," aerobic dance, or other popular classes. In fact, the workout term "aerobics" is not even a half-century old, although humans have been doing it for millions of years. In the late 1960s, Dr. Kenneth Cooper, an exercise physiologist for the San Antonio Air Force Hospital in Texas, coined the term "aerobics" to describe the system of exercise that he devised to help prevent coronary artery disease that included jogging, running, walking, and biking. His book *Aerobics* came out in 1968 and became an immediate national bestseller.

But since that time, the overfat population exploded. Billions of people became more run-down, injured, and unhealthy. While Cooper's aerobic revolution was successful on paper, it failed in practice for two reasons:

- Many people fell into overtraining through anaerobic workouts that neglected the fat-burning functions of the aerobic system.
- Junk food became popular, further impairing aerobic function.

Any workout can become anaerobic when the intensity of running, biking, dance, and other workouts is too high. While anaerobic efforts may burn more calories during the workout, the process does not train the body to specifically burn more stored fat calories over the next twenty-four hours.

It's time for a new aerobic revolution—one that's easier to implement, more practical, and with rapid-return benefits to reduce body fat.

While most people know a little bit about the muscular, hormonal, skeletal, and various other systems of the body, the full strength of the aerobic system is very rarely discussed even though it significantly influences all the others.

A powerful aerobic muscle system is a key feature of any healthy individual. The same goes for all high-performance athletes—those involved in endurance rely on it for competitive success, and strength-based athletes depend upon aerobic function to help power muscles.

Aerobic muscle fibers are the muscle cells associated with fatigue-free, fat-burning activities. They are the primary form of physical support for our joints, bones, other muscles, and essentially the entire body. Aerobic fibers are mixed into virtually all our muscles alongside smaller numbers of anaerobic fibers, which are involved in very short-term strength activity.

It's easy to perform too much anaerobic exercise. This exercise imbalance, a common result of this no-pain, no-gain philosophy of high-intensity exercise, can reduce markers

---

CAN WE BE FIT BUT UNHEALTHY?

In 2016, my colleague Professor Paul Laursen and I published an important paper in the journal *Sports Medicine*. First, we defined health and fitness differently:

Health: a state of complete, mental, social, and physical well-being, where all bodily systems (nervous, hormonal, immune, digestive, etc.) function in harmony.
Fitness: the quality of being able to perform a specific physical task, which includes exercise and sports performance.

Then, we described how exercisers, including competitive athletes, could be fit but unhealthy. An example is a person who regularly works out but is often injured, frequently ill, or has conditions such as asthma or allergies. A marathoner who dies of a heart attack mid-race is a sad example. Most of these problems are preventable. So is being overfat, despite working out many hours.

The recipe for being fit but unhealthy includes an excess amount of high training intensity or training volume and/or excess consumption of processed/refined dietary carbohydrates.

Those who exercise mistakenly believe they need more sugar for energy, and that they can "burn off" those junk food calories with more training. It's one reason why the overfat pandemic has not necessarily spared those working out regularly, including competitive athletes.

---

of health and fitness, creating damaging oxidative stress, decrease immune function, promote inflammation, damage muscles, cause fatigue, and promote posture and gait irregularity, along with reducing aerobic function and fat-burning. In short, many people who exercise, from beginners and those working out in gyms or classes to competitive athletes, actually sacrifice their health in attempting to get more fit.

NO PAIN, NO GAIN . . . NO FAT-BURNING!

One fast way to turn off our fat-burning engine is to eat junk food, a common problem both in people who work out and those who are inactive. Both of these groups share a common problem of not burning enough body fat, and poor health. The result has been an interesting but sad society-wide situation—both groups also share very similar conditions including physical injuries, depression, illness, and even heart attacks—conditions thought to be prevented by exercise. In other words, following the herd, an example of no-pain, no-gain behavior, is more likely to result in injury, disease, and burnout. That's in great part because it's more like following a diet or other cookbook recommendation, and opposite that of individuality.

The notion of no-pain, no-gain did not originate with the running boom or Jane Fonda, but actually much farther back with Benjamin Franklin.

I wrote an important article entitled "The Social Stress of 'No-Pain No-Gain'" with sociology professor Rik Scarce. We addressed the no-pain, no-gain mindset, born out of economics, and with the potential to cause undue stress. The problem is not unique to the exercise community but endemic to society as a whole. Likewise, related physical, biochemical, and mental-emotional stress conditions, from sports injuries to heart attacks, not to mention the overfat pandemic, are observed broadly across society, occurring at very similar rates in active and inactive people alike.

Benjamin Franklin was one of the early philosophers of capitalism and wrote about how to succeed in a capitalist society. As a social strain, no-pain, no-gain can tear you down, whether you're an overworked Wall Street executive, health practitioner, student, or athlete. The mechanism of burnout has reduced fat-burning and fat-storing as its base. A spiraling reduction in metabolism and overall health can lead to various physical, biochemical, and mental-emotional "injuries."

Not only is no-pain, no-gain a broad concept that applies to all of society, but it also is applied, along with unique pains and gains, to isolated groups, such as runners or other athletes, or even non-athletes. Runners and couch potatoes, for example, form distinct groups with attitudes and diverse lifestyle habits that influence how and where they fit into society. Because human behavior is sensitive to and strongly influenced by our social environment, as advertisers well know, no-pain, no-gain remains a prevalent sales pitch used to influence the general public's mental and physical health, and fitness too.

There are many examples of how no-pain, no-gain hurts us, with reduced fat-burning and the overfat pandemic being an obvious one. Here are some others:

Heart Disease
The increased risk of heart disease and death appear in both competitive athletes and otherwise similar non-athlete age groups. A 2012 study published in the *New England Journal of Medicine* looked at running events between the years 2000 and 2010 and found that of the 10.9 million runners who participated in marathons and half-marathons in the US, 59

suffered a fatal heart attack while participating, an incidence rate of 0.54 per 100,000 runners. The authors state that there is no lower incidence of sudden death in runners compared to the general population.

Asthma

According to the Centers for Disease Control and Prevention, the prevalence of asthma in the US population in 2013 was 8.3 percent in children and 7 percent in adults. By comparison, in 2012, Kippelen and colleagues collected data from athletes in the previous five summer and winter Olympic Games, showing that about 8 percent had asthma.

Depression

A 2013 study in Germany showed that the prevalence for depressive symptoms in elite athletes was 15 percent, comparable to that in the general German population.

Injuries

Mild to moderate pain-related physical injuries are the most common health problems in both athletes and non-athletes. These include sprains and strains, "pulled" muscles, joint pain, and others. Most are non-traumatic. In a given year, more than 50 percent of athletes may suffer a training-related injury, even in non-contact sports. Likewise, for those engaged in aerobic dance, group calisthenics, strength training, and those who use gym equipment. Pain is the most commonly associated symptom of these injuries. Despite the difficulty of gathering data for comparison, non-exercise-related unintentional injury rates among the general public are not dissimilar. An Institute of Medicine report states that 100 million Americans have physical pain conditions. Certainly the majority of these individuals would not be athletes or even regular exercisers. Pain is also associated with inflammation, and both are key components of virtually all injuries; sugar and other refined carbohydrates are a very common contributor of inflammation.

Overfat Athletes and Military

Some of the most popular amateur sports include running, triathlon, golf, tennis, and others. We know that today, many of these serious competitive athletes struggle with excess body fat. For those of us who have participated or watched sports for decades, the difference is quite real: both amateur and professional athletes, along with those in the military, are getting more overfat.

Consider these studies:

- The *Journal of Athletic Training* (2016) showed that the BMI of college football players increased by 38 percent from 1956 to 2014, *which significantly exceeds the rate for age-matched controls in the general population.* The authors emphasized the seriousness of the problem because of this risk factor for adverse health consequences.
- An informal survey from *Golf Digest* claims that two-thirds of recreational golfers are overweight. No surprise here, and this is the same rate as the American population, which could mean that the number of overfat golfers is closer to 90 percent.
- A 2016 study in the journal *Obesity Research & Clinical Practice* examined 145 years of data on body mass in 17,918 male professional baseball players in the US. It showed that for 120 years, most baseball players were classified as normal weight and almost none were obese.

But in the past 25 years, 70 percent are now overweight, and 10 percent are obese, with only 20 percent of professional baseball players being normal weight. Some of these normal-weight players are no doubt also overfat.

The military also has an interest in body composition due to its relation with physical performance. The *Military Times* (September 2016) says "Today's military is fatter than ever." They report that the number of overweight and obese US men and women has roughly doubled during the past five years and is up fourfold since 2001. In the US Army, for example, as of 2011, 52 percent of service members were considered overweight, with 16 percent obese. A 2015 study in the journal *Preventive Medicine Reports* states that army soldiers who were overweight and obese with increased muscle mass also had disproportionate increases in fat—they had higher BMIs due to more body fat as opposed to lean body mass.

A healthy increase in muscle mass can help performance in certain professional athletes, such as in football, and those in the military. However, being overfat and muscular can adversely impact fitness, while significantly impairing current and future health. Specifically, overfat and fit individuals can have reductions in important performance functions: running speed and endurance, agility and flexibility, cardiovascular responsiveness and recovery, and resistance to illness and injury.

In many ways, we are only as healthy as the world around us, with social influences affecting our behavior and habits regardless of whether one is an athlete or couch potato. It's the reason worker wellness programs are still unsuccessful most of the time—the spectrum of people who make up large and small companies are a part of the same unhealthy society. A particular wellness program may influence individual people, but as a whole, a group of workers is also a reflection of society.

We are a society of aerobic beings. This is how our individual bodies have worked since the beginning. Our hunter-gatherer routines involved a lot of fat-burning—walking and easy running to find and collect food, with the occasional sprint to escape being eaten. Unfortunately, problematic social trends such as "no pain, no gain" and the popularity and addiction to junk food have impaired aerobic function in the majority of people on earth. The result has been a serious, ongoing problem called aerobic deficiency syndrome, which affects billions of people.

EXERCISE DEPENDENCE: POSITIVE ADDICTION OR DECEPTIVE DISORDER?

Are you preoccupied with working out? If you miss a day, or more, are there withdrawal symptoms such as that of depression or physically just not right? Do you still train if you're hurt or sick? Do you try to squeeze workouts in during lunch or sacrifice sleep time for it? Does exercise interfere with personal relationships, work, or social responsibilities? If some of these factors are part of your life you could have an addiction known as *exercise dependence*.

Too much of a good thing is not a new concept. It was Hippocrates who first said that everything in excess is opposed to nature. The term exercise dependence describes people who continue exercising when socially or medically contraindicated, when it interferes with relationships and work, and when missing a day or more produces withdrawal symptoms. Among the problems with this disorder is that the stress it creates can impair fat-burning, and if it's extreme it can cause a serious loss of body fat.

The academic discussion of excessive physical activity often focuses on obsessive and compulsive exercising. Researchers say the most appropriate term for this phenomenon is exercise addiction, emphasizing that excessive physical exercise fits the typical and most common characteristics of behavioral addictions. Other terms have also been used such as exercise abuse and compulsive exercise. Mild, less defined, functional versions of exercise dependence would be much more common. Regardless of the names and where one falls on the spectrum, an exercise disorder can be considered part of the overtraining syndrome.

A behavioral addiction can potentially be observed in anyone who works out, from competitive athletes on all levels driven to improve performances to casual exercisers driven to lose weight or improve body image. In many cases, these individuals may also demonstrate another common clinical problem previously discussed: disordered eating. If the "drive" to workout becomes an *overdrive*, the brain's HPA axis (hypothalamic-pituitary-adrenal) can lead to physical, biochemical, or mental-emotional harm.

The concept of *exercise dependence* first appeared in the medical journals following the running boom of the 1970s, which soon included walkers, cyclists, triathletes, and others. The risk of exercise dependency increases when individuals follow the guise of more is better (a.k.a. "no-pain, no-gain").

While some research estimates rates of exercise dependence are very high with others showing it's very low, depending on the types of exercisers and specific definitions, rates for competitive endurance athletes may range between 25 and 50 percent.

In 1976, psychiatrist William Glasser's book *Postitive Addiction* became a hit, in particular with many runners who could relate to being addicted to their sport. However, Glasser was not writing about the potential for exercise dependency. He defined "positive addiction" as something non-competitive, easy to do, performed alone most times, and that the activity must be done without self-criticism. This was not a common profile of many athletes during this period, and even today.

Other researchers would not accept "addiction" as being associated with something positive, arguing that the symptoms of addiction should only be applied to unhealthy exercise behavior. This would involve workouts leading to frequent and sometimes serious injuries, to not just knees and ankles, but hearts and heads too. The stress of training and racing, for example, can sometimes lead to depression and anxiety. Heart attacks were not normal either.

Writing in the journal *Mayo Clinic Proceedings* ("Exercising for Health and Longevity vs Peak Performance: Different Regimens for Different Goals," September 2014), authors O'Keefe, Franklin, and Lavie state that, "'Cardiac overuse injury' is the term we have suggested for this increasingly common consequence of the 'more exercise is better' strategy." They highlight various studies that basically infer that many athletes are fit but unhealthy, including, in distance runners for example, increased risk of atrial fibrillation, high levels of coronary artery plaque, and the annual report of heart attacks during races. In some cases, those who train at higher volumes and intensities are at even higher risk than sedentary individuals.

The story is clear, as is the research: exercise can potentially, significantly, contribute to better physical, biochemical, and mental-emotional health, which includes tuning your metabolism to be better at fat-burning. However, this is not true of either extreme—a sedentary lifestyle or overtraining.

How much of a good thing can turn bad? Of course, it's all about balancing both health and fitness, and recognizing imbalance in its earliest stages as a key to preventing it.

Through the years there have been many physiological and psychological theories about how one becomes addicted to exercise, but without consensus. One factor is certain—society and its influence on individuals plays a major role, in part by creating misconceptions about exercise (much like diet) encouraging these negative behaviors.

When it comes to the health benefits of exercise, numerous studies emphasize a conservative approach to working out, especially if some high-intensity training is included in one's routine. For example, a schedule of fewer than five hours a week of working out may be the safe upper range for long-term cardiovascular and metabolic benefits. In addition, two days off from exercise, and refraining from daily high-intensity exercise can help maintain a good balance of health and fitness.

In the large and long-term Copenhagen City Heart Study (*Journal of the American College of Cardiology*, February 2015) it was shown that low and moderate intensity runners had a lower mortality compared to that of sedentary people, but those training at high intensities had a mortality rate not statistically different from the sedentary group. The authors concluded that the benefits of running "are most robust for those who jog between 1 and 2.5 h per week, at a slow to moderate pace, at a frequency of about 2 or 3 times per week."

Does this mean we can't train enough to develop our full athletic potentials? Certainly not. The real game at this high level of sports performance is avoiding crossing into overtraining where there are negative consequences—a game too many competitive athletes lose, as indicated by physical, biochemical, and mental-emotional injuries.

We can train for optimal competition in a healthy way without the excesses. This is accomplished by building the aerobic system to burn more fat by moderating volume, balancing intensity, eating well, and managing stress. In short, an unhealthy body won't tolerate higher volumes and or intensities.

In the case of professional athletes, we can push the envelope more because these individuals are cared for more closely (or should be), thereby better adapting to the stresses of training, fine-tuning their physical bodies, determining their precise nutritional needs, and so on. (This can certainly be accomplished with any individual if the same lifestyle factors and health-care support are incorporated successfully.)

In general, our lifestyle either promotes health . . . or it does not. Yet the details sometimes become fuzzy and we have to figure those out. If we second-guess our motives because we read or hear about other approaches, like the latest diet or workout craze, it can easily get us off course.

THE AEROBIC DEFICIENCY SYNDROME

With most of the world overfat, aerobic deficiency is common. It can develop quickly from eating junk food, from too little physical activity, or from over-emphasizing high-intensity training, and can affect everyone from couch potatoes to professional athletes. Some of the signs and symptoms associated with aerobic deficiency include:

- Chronic fatigue
- Physical injury
- Poor endurance
- Hormone imbalance
- Chronic inflammation
- Pain
- Hunger (including during or after exercise)
- Reduced fat-burning
- Increased body fat

TRUE AEROBIC ACTIVITY

Common activities such as running, biking, swimming, dancing, and walking can be *either* aerobic or anaerobic, depending on the intensity of the workout. While this can be measured in a laboratory, the easiest way to monitor each exercise session to ensure aerobic development is by checking your heart rate. Lower heart rate exercise can build the aerobic system and burn more body fat—as long as you avoid junk food.

Your heart rate is an accurate indicator of intensity—lower heart rate exercise tends to be aerobic, while performing the same workout with a higher heart rate would be anaerobic. This does not mean you will always be slow: building the aerobic system allows the body to move faster over time, and at the same heart rate. Walkers, runners, cyclists, and others will get faster over time with the same heart rate and level of effort.

This is where the issues get more complicated. In the short term, almost any activity—even very hard efforts—can help temporarily build the aerobic muscles. But continue these kinds of exercise routines for too long and your aerobic system can break down through overtraining. You may become injured and fatigued, and your health may suffer because you are pursuing fitness at the expense of health. Instead, the best approach is to first build a great aerobic system.

Without a great aerobic system, it could take a period of three to six months or more to specifically develop it. During this period of time it's important to avoid high-intensity exercise.

A true aerobic workout should feel relatively easy initially. Some say it feels too easy, but that just reflects the level of your aerobic system—those with poor aerobic function, and poor fat-burning, are unable to move very fast. But once the aerobic muscles begin developing and more energy is derived from fat, activities increase at the same level of intensity, the same heart rate.

When you've finished each aerobic workout, you should feel great—not tired or sore, and certainly not ready to collapse on the couch. You should almost feel you can do the same workout again. Nor should you crave sugar or other carbohydrates; aerobic workouts program your body to burn stored fat, not sugar. To make sure you are attaining all the benefits of aerobic exercise, determine the heart rate best for your individual needs using my 180-Formula.

THE 180-FORMULA: HELPING YOU TAKE THE GUESSWORK OUT OF AEROBIC EXERCISE

To find your maximum aerobic training heart rate, there are two important steps. First, subtract your age from 180. Next, find the best category for your present state of fitness and health, and make the appropriate adjustments:

1. Subtract your age from 180.
2. Modify this number by selecting among the following categories the one that best matches your fitness and health profile:
    a. If you have or are recovering from a major illness (heart disease, any operation or hospital stay, etc.) or are on any regular medication, subtract an additional 10.
    b. If you are injured, have regressed in training or competition, get more than two colds or bouts of flu per year, have allergies or asthma, or if you have been inconsistent or are just getting back into training, subtract an additional 5.
    c. If you have been training consistently (at least four times weekly) for up to two years without any of the problems just mentioned, keep the number (180 minus age) the same.
    d. If you have been training for more than two years without any of the problems listed above, and have made progress in competition without injury, add 5.

For example, if you are thirty years old and fit into category (b), you get the following:

180–30=150. Then 150–5=145 beats per minute (bpm).

In this example, 145 will be the highest heart rate for all training. This is highly aerobic, allowing you to most efficiently build an aerobic base. Training above this heart rate rapidly incorporates anaerobic function, exemplified by a shift to burning more sugar and less fat for fuel.

If it is difficult to decide which of two groups best fits you, choose the group or outcome that results in the lower heart rate. In athletes who are taking medication that may affect their heart rate, those who wear a pacemaker, or those who have special circumstances not discussed here, further individualization with the help of a health-care practitioner or other specialist familiar with your circumstance and knowledgeable in endurance sports may be necessary.

For competitive athletes, two situations may be exceptions to the above calculations:

- The 180-Formula may need to be further individualized for athletes over the age of sixty-five. Up to 10 beats may have to be added for those only in category (d) in the 180-Formula, and depending on individual levels of fitness and health. This does not mean 10 should automatically be added, but that an honest self-assessment is important.
- For athletes sixteen years of age and under, the formula is not applicable; rather, a heart rate of 165 may be best.

Once a maximum aerobic heart rate is found, a range from this heart rate to 10 beats below could be used for training. For example, if an athlete's maximum aerobic heart rate is determined to be 155, that person's aerobic training zone would be 145 to 155 bpm. However, the more training that person does at 155, the quicker an optimal aerobic base will be developed. The use of a heart rate monitor is the most accurate way to ensure you avoid exceeding your maximum aerobic rate.

HOW MONITORING YOUR HEART RATE HELPS BURN FAT

We call devices that measure heart rate "heart-rate monitors," but you could also call them "fat-burning monitors" since monitoring your pulse rate during exercise is the best way to promote fat-burning both during and after your workout.

Unfortunately, in our no-pain, no-gain world, some people use heart-rate monitors improperly—to push themselves even harder, and to see how high their heart rate will go.

A heart-rate monitor is a basic biofeedback device. With correct use, it can help you regulate the workout so you build a great aerobic system.

Reducing excess body fat is best accomplished by avoiding junk food and eating healthy foods. True aerobic exercise can enhance these fat-burning benefits, along with many other health and fitness improvements.

COMPETITIVE ATHLETES CAN TEST AEROBIC IMPROVEMENT

As the aerobic system develops, increased fat-burning brings more speed and power. Testing yourself with a heart monitor can help evaluate whether you are indeed on the right track. It allows you to more objectively measure improvements in workouts. Instead of hoping exercise is giving you benefits only to find that weeks or months later not much has changed, a simple evaluation can be performed. As we burn more body fat, aerobic muscle function improves and you will be able to walk or run with more speed, bike with more power, or otherwise improve performance at the same heart rate. This is especially important for competitive athletes, as training paces predict race paces. This evaluation is called the maximum aerobic function (MAF) test. Below is an example of a runner's improved pace at the same aerobic heart rate over time.

	April	May	June	July
Mile time:	8:21	8:11	7:57	7:44

For more details about this and other athletic training information, see my *Big Book of Endurance Training and Racing*.

CHAPTER 9

AN OVERFAT ECONOMY

POOR HEALTH MAKES MANY PEOPLE RICH

Health care is big business. It has grown alongside the overfat pandemic during the past few decades. The reason? Being overfat makes people sick, leading to the need for more health-care products and services. It's a simple matter of supply and demand.

We don't really have a health-care system—it's disease care, and one that is among the most successful revenue-generating industries in history. The system discourages people from getting healthy by addressing symptoms instead of treating the causes of illness, and by keeping the elderly alive longer, a period when medical costs usually soar.

Do the powers-that-be want to change this? It's a goose laying golden eggs.

But what if enough people took charge of their health and reduced excess body fat, thus reducing health-care costs? At least initially, a shift from disease care to true health care would bring a devastating economic shift not only in the US but around the globe.

Most individuals are concerned about their health-care costs, from insurance premiums to deductibles and out-of-pocket expenses. Many also watch the economy because of its effects on their personal financial securities and cost of living. The stock market is not only where many people save for retirement, but it significantly affects the overall economy.

With health-care stocks booming in the long run, most experts think they are poised to continue, that is, unless something unforeseen happens. That something could be enough people getting healthy quickly to the point of tipping the balance of supply and demand. This could drop stocks. A collapse in share prices has the potential to cause widespread economic disruption.

OVERFAT ECONOMICS

The economies of most countries are such that governments spend more money on health care than any other programs—in the US it's more than military, education, and even much more than running the government itself.

The rapid and continuous rise in health-care costs are in great part due to the overfat pandemic that has quietly exploded. It's left massive numbers of casualties, people with preventable diseases and disabilities whose costs are out of control. It was President Theodore Roosevelt who said, "No country can be strong whose people are sick and poor."

In 2015, US health-care expenses, which includes federal and state governments, individuals and businesses, grew almost 6 percent from the previous year to $3.2 trillion (compare this to the US military budget of about $575 million). Health care accounted for almost 18 percent of the gross domestic product, with the estimates for 2017 to be 22 percent.

To put the 2015 numbers into perspective, $3.2 trillion is nearly $10,000 per person; that's almost $40,000 a year for a family of four, while the median household income of this family the same year was just over $56,000.

Prescription drug spending alone was the fastest growth area, increasing 9 percent to nearly $325 billion in 2015.

Wall Street's health-care sector houses health-care providers and services, equipment and supply companies, and the related biotechnology and pharmaceutical industries. Stock prices have been booming for many years. Although a bit down in 2016, some see this as a buying opportunity with estimations for great growth for 2017. Analysts on "the Street" expect health-care stocks to keep booming, claiming the long-term track record of consistent outperformance is likely to continue because demands for health-care products and services keep rising, especially with the growth of adult diseases in children and an aging population. The growing overfat pandemic has, and will, continue to fuel these money-making ventures. But is this sustainable?

It is, as long as poor health makes many people rich. But it's not if something is done to improve population health.

That something is *you*. It's *us*. If enough individuals take charge and manage their health—and are even only moderately successful—it could reduce disease-care spending significantly. It could also lead to the bursting of one of the biggest bubbles in Wall Street history, crashing the entire stock market and economy.

But we'll recover, and could be healthier for it.

THE OVERFAT ECONOMY

The stark reality is that the US leads the world's direction in health and sickness. The US has higher rates of overall mortality, and both premature and preventable death, of all industrialized countries, who are not far behind. All while the US spends the most on health care. Developing nations, who are already experiencing serious levels of overfat, are catching up too.

There is an illusion that modern health care improves aging and quality of life, but the truth is that today's longer lifespan is just a smokescreen. People aren't living longer so much as they are just dying slower. The costs are wrecking world economy, and we already can't afford it.

We have now created a big chunk of our economy based on the overfat pandemic, complete with high rates of diseases that are not cheap to diagnose and treat. And, dysfunctional aging will continue to worsen with rising rates of seniors; the average American survives more than a decade of infirmity before death, running up untold billions of dollars in care.

Rising rates of Alzheimer's, diabetes, cardiovascular disorders, and cancer grab the headlines. However, the unacceptable rates of those who are overfat constitutes the real underlying problem, one mostly untreated, that leads to these diseases.

Even many of those who have given up smoking cigarettes and gotten off the couch to regularly exercise, two important lifestyle changes, are still overfat, continually fueling higher rates of disease.

Amid all this disease and dysfunction, the fact that expensive and profitable high-tech medicine can keep unhealthy people living longer than ever still creates the illusion that our health-care system is working. But consider these facts:

- With the highest rates of disease burden, the US ranks first in the word in Disability Adjusted Life Years (DALYs), a measure of premature deaths and the number of years lost to disability.
- America ranks thirty-seventh in the World Health Organization's international ranking of health systems (Cuba is close behind at thirty-ninth, and with recent political changes could catch us). Yet the US ranks first in health expenditure, a position we won't lose too soon.
- At around 20 percent of the US gross domestic product, the highest of all developed nations and still climbing, health-care costs remain a significant drag on the economy.
- A mere 3,300 junk food industry lobbyists, give or take, are fighting to keep these costs rising by continuing to encourage the consumption of bad food.

What if all this changed?

What if individuals took control to manage their own health? And what if this resulted in health-care costs being reduced by 50 percent within 12 months?

Is this really possible? Yes.

Over the last 40 years, I have witnessed this decline in individual health-care expense through my work with thousands of patients. In fact, 50 percent in 12 months is a poor response, as most people improve health significantly much sooner, with health-care expenses reducing more than 50 percent.

In chapter 6, I referred to a study demonstrating that the majority of children tested reversed chronic metabolic disease indicators, such as high levels of cholesterol, high blood pressure, high blood sugar and insulin, liver dysfunction, and other problems, *in just ten days* by giving up foods with added sugars. Numerous other studies demonstrate that low-carbohydrate eating can quickly improve many risk factors such as hypertension, high blood cholesterol (total and LDL), high blood triglycerides, high glucose and insulin, and others. Reducing these markers in adults and children means less medication, fewer doctor visits, less frequent disease, and ultimately less money spent.

Most health-care dollars go toward treating preventable conditions that were not prevented, despite the cost of prevention being very cheap. Prevention through self-health management would involve individuals making healthier choices. Based on how easily and quickly this can happen, a dramatic turnaround of health care can really happen, and soon.

While the US leads the way in being overfat, with high rates of heart disease and cancer, and many other measures of

---

A HEALTHY AMERICA, A HEALTHY WORLD

The US leads the world in many innovations, inventions, technology, and other modern developments that make the world a better place. But America also leads the world in being overfat. While some countries leapfrogged over US levels during the explosion of the overfat pandemic, it was the US that blazed the trail.

Now, the US can blaze a new trail, by reducing the overfat pandemic. We know how to do this—the real question is how long it will take to implement.

While a consensus exists about the dangers of junk foods causing the overfat pandemic, the issue of what to do about it too

---

often becomes a game. It's unnecessarily complicated, with government agencies and some scientists saying "more research is needed." And while the research is being done, the overfat pandemic continues to worsen. As a country or as a planet, we never get to implement the remedies that small but rising numbers of clinicians have used successfully for generations.

As powerful as self-health management is, here are some of the well-documented scientific strategies that governments can implement. These can help accomplish a population-wide reduction in the overfat pandemic even quicker, triggering dramatic reductions in disease and health-care expenses:

- Widespread public education campaigns.
- Revised food labels to call attention to added sugar.
- Adding warning labels to sugar-sweetened products.
- Increased nutrition education for health-care providers.
- Increased education early in school (and implementing healthy cafeteria food).
- Banning the sale of refined carbohydrates, including beverages (such as sports drinks, energy drinks, and sodas) in schools, at school-related events, and in hospitals.
- Banning the advertising of refined carbohydrates.
- The taxing of refined carbohydrate foods, including foods with added sugar.
- Prohibition of government subsidies associated with refined carbohydrates.

If some of these recommendations sound familiar, or even appear extreme, there is precedence. These are very similar to those applied to alcohol and tobacco long ago. Such changes could contribute substantially to reducing population-wide intake of junk food, leading to substantial improvement in public health.

Unfortunately, while this is the direction we are headed, politics will prevent the rapid action, taking many years to implement these changes. During this time the overfat pandemic will keep growing, and more people will have a significantly lower quality of life, develop disease, and die slowly. This is not acceptable. Why wait? *You* can manage your own health now to make these changes happen almost overnight.

poor health, a shift to a healthier America could start a new trend: a healthy world.

IT'S THE SUGAR, STUPID

During Bill Clinton's successful 1992 presidential campaign, he stated, "the economy, stupid." In other words, sometimes the simplest solutions are staring us in the face.

There is a scientific consensus that poor food quality is one of our major risk factors associated with disease and poor quality of life. The worst health habits that contribute most to chronic disease have been outlined by the World Health Organization (WHO). These are associated with:

- Bad food
- Inactivity
- Tobacco use
- Alcohol excess

The WHO claims that eliminating these problems could lead to at least an 80 percent reduction of all heart disease, stroke, and type 2 diabetes, along with high rates of cancer. This is in line with my clinical observations.

But *this* probably won't happen. Health care is too political and too big a business.

"Follow the money" was the famous catchphrase popularized by the 1976 movie *All the President's Men*. It suggests a corrupt, political money trail that led to the Watergate scandal. A very similar but bigger scandal exists with Big Sugar and governments around the world, one that started long before Watergate, and continues today.

Addressing bad food, *and* exercise, *and* smoking, *and* alcohol excess, with the stronghold of politics and business means these changes won't happen too soon. How can we sort through all this to simplify the remedy?

I recall one of my first patients, who had a variety of complaints, including some serious chronic problems. Feeling the devastating effects of poor aging, he said he'd do anything to be healthy again. After evaluating him, and his lifestyle habits, I gave him a comprehensive report, including recommendations I knew would reverse his poor health and make him feel young again. It included:

- Improving his diet, providing details about the healthy balance of carbohydrates, fats, and proteins, the need to eat a lot of vegetables, and the importance of avoiding skipping meals during his busy workday.
- A simple exercise program, with a variety of options.
- The need to quit smoking was obvious, so I offered a number of programs that had good success, and the possible option of quitting *cold turkey*.
- Finally, I suggested he reduce the consumption of alcohol from three to four drinks a day to a moderate level of two.

I was proud of my thorough assessment process and comprehensive report. My patient thanked me several times before leaving the clinic.

Needless to say, I never heard from him again. He was overwhelmed and overloaded with healthy recommendations. Regardless whether they were going to be effective or not, the plan was doomed to fail before it started.

Learning an important lesson forced me to change my approach. Instead of overwhelming patients by presenting the details of every helpful lifestyle change, recommendations were simplified. I would present the most powerful and important single recommendation—the primary problem that could change health quickly and most significantly was the starting point. In most cases, it was eliminating refined carbohydrates.

This was not the recommendation for *everyone*, as it's not a one-size-fits-all approach. Some patients had acute pain and required immediate care, some were athletes who sought coaching, and still others were more complicated cases. However, forty years ago, the consumption of junk food was widespread, and the explosion of the overfat pandemic already had begun. Many people were experiencing the adverse effects of refined carbohydrates, even if they were not overweight or obese.

I soon learned that those patients who would give up sugar and other junk food improved their health more significantly and faster than others. Sure, people still needed to moderate alcohol, exercise properly, and not smoke. But these habit changes would come later, and much easier once carbohydrate intolerance was no longer a devastating problem.

The overwhelming consensus among scientists and clinicians, at least those without conflicts of interest, is that bad food choices lead to poor health—and healthy eating habits can improve and very quickly reverse it. Simple.

THE ONE-SIZE-FITS-ALL ECONOMY

We've come to expect government and health-care agencies to tell us how to eat. They've been promoting their guidelines for decades, all while the world got overfat. But one-size dietary recommendations don't fit everyone. Low-carb, ketogenic, low-fat, hi-lo-whatever is just sales hype. It might make good economic sense if you're a seller, but for consumers it's an insult. The one-size-fits-all economy has wrecked our health and produced the overfat pandemic.

In addition, billions of big-business research dollars are spent trying to understand why people are overfat. Whenever a researcher gets close to showing how certain dietary components influence insulin or body fat, these ideas are not implemented because the game is to state that "more research is needed." In other words, "we're not sure yet, so give us more research money." This is great ammunition for Big Sugar, who keeps claiming there is no research to confirm that sugar is unhealthy, and keeps politicians from implementing useful, updated policies directed at improving the health of their populations (especially considering that Big Sugar lobbies overshadow them). If you're among the sheep, the herd is headed for the cliff.

But we're individuals taking charge of our own health, and enough of us can change our own health and the economic mess we're all in. We can be rewarded for our due diligence. Without this approach, the ongoing confusion continues about getting and staying healthy, especially when it comes to reducing excess body fat.

As is well-known, insulin is strongly associated with body fat—too much of the former can contribute to the latter. The many downstream problems associated with this common cause include chronic diseases such as type 2 diabetes, cancer, cardiovascular diseases, and many others that are devastating the economy. The pharmaceutical industry knows this—drugs that reduce insulin also reduce body fat. But this is not the only answer, as lifestyle changes can do the same—you just have to know which eating pattern works for your body's

LIFESTYLE FACTORS THAT PROMOTE INCREASED INSULIN AND BODY FAT

Besides junk food, other lifestyle factors can increase body fat. They include genetics, the number of beta-cells in the pancreas, and other factors we have little or no control over. Excess stress can also be a factor. But for most people, food is the most influential factor. While micronutrients, vitamins, and minerals affect the insulin–body fat process, the macronutrients are the most dominant food factor:

Fat: dietary fat can sometimes, in some individuals, increase insulin, often in the presence of carbohydrates. A diet too high in fat and carbohydrate may be the most common way billions of people eat, and certainly a reason why up to 76 percent of the world is overfat. Eating only natural fats and carbohydrates is key.

Protein: too much dietary protein can increase insulin stimulation too, and if so can increase fat storage. The most influential amino acids in this regard are arginine, and the so-called branched-chain amino acids—isoleucine, leucine, valine, tyrosine, and phenylalanine. The problems can sometimes be in the use of dietary supplements of these amino acids, or the dependence on high-protein diets. Eating moderate amounts of concentrated protein foods work best, choosing from eggs, dairy, and meats.

Carbohydrate: whether in combination with fat and/or protein, carbohydrate foods are the most powerful stimulator of insulin and contributor to increased body fat. Avoiding junk food in all its disguises remains rule number one, not only if you want to reduce excess body fat but for overall improved health and fitness, too.

There are plenty of studies that demonstrate how fat, protein, and carbohydrate influence insulin, body fat storage, and poor health, although most are on the carb-insulin connection. These usually have cautious results that often appear conflicting because there is clearly considerable variability in the relative responses to these foods between individuals. Yes, we all respond a bit differently to food. Unfortunately, no study has simultaneously compared the responsiveness to dietary fat, protein, and carbohydrate.

fat-burning need. Obviously, drugs come with side effects, are expensive, and don't address the cause of the problem—eating junk food. And lifestyle changes are essentially free.

Because carbohydrate foods immediately influence insulin to increase body fat storage, it's the best place to start to make healthy changes for most people. It's why I developed the Two-Week Test—as a way to do our very own research, a study of one.

Our variability in response to food is one of the human features we possess that makes us uniquely different from each other. While researchers claim that genetic profiling studies will soon help us understand the mechanistic underpinnings of this variation—our individual responses to food—and usher in a new era of *nutrigenomics* to prevent excess body fat and disease, we don't really have to wait. We can already do this by taking charge of our health.

Individualization is the only real proof in human health studies. It's the study of one. While usually taken as an excuse for why things *don't* work, the scientific approach of looking for the answer really means searching for that one-size-fits-all remedy, and when it's not found it leads to the notion that more research is needed. We already possess what we're looking for.

MORE ECONOMIC NEWS

Junk food kills, even if you are profiting from it. Simply not eating junk food is a logical remedy and alternative to the current unaffordable state of poor health. But business begs to differ, with ongoing multimillion-dollar marketing campaigns by Big Sugar directed at adults and children on all socioeconomic levels, keeping our world on the road to ill health and rising health-care spending. (This is not unlike Big Tobacco's campaigns of the 1950s and '60s, when even doctors were paid to promote the so-called benefits of smoking.)

Two economic-based articles have recently focused on this issue:

- The International Diabetes Federation urged the G20 (of the world's major advanced and emerging economies), which met in Turkey in 2015, to cooperate in fighting obesity in the same way as they acted together in the 2008 financial crisis. Some countries, including Mexico, Chile, and France, have already experimented with different variations of sugar taxation, but there are considerable political obstacles, as well as resistance from the food industry.

- Credit Suisse, a large multinational financial services company, published an article, "Is Sugar Turning the Economy Sour?," in late 2013 that highlighted some of the same economic issues described here. In a corresponding study led by Stefano Natella, head of Global Equity Research at Credit Suisse, called "Sugar: Consumption at a crossroads," it found that close to 90 percent of general practitioners surveyed in the US, Europe, and Asia believe excess sugar consumption is linked to the sharp growth in diabetes and obesity. In referring to the health problems associated with sugar consumption, the authors stated that, "we cannot ignore the significance and the implications for society and our economy any longer."

There's no doubt that both long- and short-term benefits can come with one simple change in food intake. But what will this mean for the economy? What would happen to the

American disease-care system if millions were to adopt this self-health approach?

Sales of prescription and over-the-counter medications would plummet. The need for wide ranges of medical services would dramatically diminish. Many businesses might disappear, especially fast-food restaurants and candy stores. Cereal sales would plummet. So would many stocks. The bubble that's been building would burst.

Transitioning to healthy America might trigger a healthier world, while killing our health-care economy.

However, the process would be one of transition, causing a shift to a new economic base. People would still spend money on food, but make better choices. Less money would be spent on prescription and over-the-counter medications, while many people—suddenly leaner—would have to buy new clothes. While fast-food chains would lose millions of customers, healthy items like fresh fruits, vegetables, meats, and eggs would divert dollars to family farms and farm stands, with many supermarkets and restaurants surviving because they would offer truly healthy foods.

The remedy is realistic and simple. It may invoke pain for some consumers, temporarily overcoming sugar addiction, and economic pains. But in the end, we could win the health-care battle.

Each one of us can be responsible for our own health by avoiding junk food in all its disguises, thereby having a higher quality of life with very low medical expenses, reduced disease risk, and more productivity. If this sounds like too much of a storybook ending or Hollywood-ish, it's not. I've witnessed it my whole career, and I've been through it myself. And if it means we have to adjust our economy and rid the world of unhealthy business, we do that too. We want the highest quality of life for as long as we can have it.

CHAPTER 10

AGING AND THE OVERFAT- UNDERFAT PARADOX

The lean and ageless Hall of Fame baseball pitcher Satchel Paige said it best: "How old would you be if you didn't know how old you were?" Too many people would say they feel or seem older than they are. If that is the case, change it!

Body fat quality and quantity are closely associated with healthy aging. Too much or too little body fat in particular can impair our health, especially as we age. This problem has developed into a paradox: a rapid transition by many overfat people to an underfat state.

WHEN OVERFAT TURNS TO UNDERFAT

One common feature of aging is that chronic disease can contribute to muscle wasting, which is also associated with the rapid and unhealthy loss of body fat. This is often seen as a transition from an overfat state to one of underfat. Both are serious unhealthy conditions, and both are preventable.

Who is *underfat*? We think of the problem of too little body fat as being associated with malnutrition, usually starvation; it's still a serious disorder, especially in developing nations. Today, for the first time in human history, the number of people who are obese far exceeds those who are underweight.

During the explosion of the overfat pandemic over the last four decades, the proportion of underweight adults globally fell from about 14 percent to about 9 percent. Unfortunately, large numbers of people within these same countries also experienced rapidly rising levels of overfat people as well, sometimes even within the same family.

Two other groups of people are underfat, a more prominent problem in Western societies where life expectancy is longer:

- Older individuals with chronic illness. The condition of sarcopenia, the loss of muscle, which can lead to sarcopenic obesity, can often end in another condition called *cachexia*. The results include a significant loss of both muscle and a state of underfat. Cachexia is a serious problem, and is present in 30 percent of patients worldwide who die—a major contributor to death worldwide. Our aging population will see this group of people rise in number significantly in the coming years.
- Those with serious eating disorders, which may be up to 70 million people globally, including those who exercise excessively, a condition called *anorexia athletica*. As the world becomes more Westernized, many more people

will start exercising and participating in sports competition, with disordered eating increasing as well, as a separate problem or one combined with exercise. The numbers of these underfat conditions can rise as well.

The overfat-underfat paradox includes another twist. In addition to the rising overfat pandemic, and the growing numbers of underfat people with chronic disease and disordered eating, the result could be a decreasing number of healthy people on the planet. My colleagues and I present this dilemma in our paper, "Overfat and Underfat: New Terms and Definitions Long Overdue."

INFLUENCE YOUR AGE

We can always strive to be younger. While we know that most debilitating chronic illnesses are preventable, including heart disease, cancer, and Alzheimer's, so is poor aging.

Larger numbers of today's elderly are living longer through heroic measures such as heart, lung, and liver transplants, around the clock care, and other medical means. For most, those "extra years" come at the end of the lifespan, not when we're young and vibrant but when life is less vigorous and productive. We can significantly control what may be the most important factor of aging—quality of life. And the sooner we start, the better.

All humans do it. The months and years pass and we get less efficient with our bodies and brains. We slow down, and it happens whether we are couch potatoes or retired Olympians. There is no stopping it—anti-aging is a myth. We can, however, significantly control the pace at which aging occurs by being healthier and more fit.

The difference is *physiological* versus *chronological* aging. This means we control aging to a great degree by choosing a lifestyle that allows us to be more like an average forty-year-old even if we were born fifty years earlier, or a forty-five-year-old even though our driver's license says 1953. Chronological age refers to the years that have passed. But when we are healthier and more fit, we function like someone younger. That is our physiological age. It's related to better blood sugar regulation, brainpower, endurance and strength, and other lifestyle features we can influence, including our posture, gait, and how we physically move.

Maintaining a healthy level of body fat, in quality and quantity, is a key part of healthy aging. Preparing for it starts at birth, and certainly is influenced by choices we make throughout our earlier life.

Modern medicine has given us many miracles, and many people would not be alive today if not for these technologies and other new developments. Oftentimes, though, these people are experiencing what is known as the prolonged dying processes. We've seen it in a grandmother, uncle, parent, or other person. And we never get used to it.

The good news is that much of our quality of life throughout the aging process is under our control, including our influence on the *preventable* diseases most people in the developed world die from: Alzheimer's, stroke, cancer, diabetes, and heart disease. These are among the diseases associated with carbohydrate intolerance.

Early in the book I highlighted three key recommendations to correct and prevent being overfat, while improving health and fitness.

- The first was to stop eating junk food.

- The second was to determine your particular level of carbohydrate intolerance, using the Two-Week Test.
- Now it's time for the third: keeping up with the carbohydrate intolerance that often worsens with age—if we don't, we can get older fast. Accomplishing this is done by making simple adjustments in food intake as the years go by.

Basically, most people become more insulin-resistant as they age—more carbohydrate intolerant. This occurs at different paces depending on the individual. Some avoid this for many years due to a great lifestyle, while others pass through the subclinical stages of carbohydrate intolerance and into the disease state, such as diabetes, by midlife. Still others experience this much earlier.

Recall the common signs and symptoms of CI, which includes sleepiness or lack of concentration after meals, intestinal bloating and gas, increases in body fat, especially in the belly, making clothes fit tighter, and perhaps most importantly, frequent hunger. While these were discussed in relation to the post-Two-Week Test activity, they are really very good indications that you are eating more carbohydrate foods than you can tolerate, that you are becoming more carbohydrate intolerant, or, as often happens, both.

When these signs and symptoms begin to appear—and the sooner you notice them and respond, the better—the remedy is simple. Reduce carbohydrate foods further until these problems disappear. For many people, performing the Two-Week Test again is a valuable exercise. Others can rely on intuition to make the appropriate adjustments. Making these changes throughout life is important. When we reach our seventies, eighties, nineties—and beyond—we want to make sure we follow the same healthy paths, even if others are shopping and preparing food for us.

AGING YOUR WAY—TO THE END

With all your dedication to reducing body fat leading to improved health, fitness, and quality of life, death is also something we all should consider. It may seem odd to be reading about this issue here, but as we age, eating right for our body should also be maintained. Assuring this will happen is an important issue to address *now*. It means talking to family members and health-care practitioners—conversations that lead to legal documentation. These might be detailed in a health-care proxy, living will, and advance directive created by legal experts.

This is especially important to maintain better brain function despite a loss of body function.

We know how we want to live, and the same should be true with dying. Death should not be an unmentionable topic, but something to discuss with our loved ones and/or legal advisor. Specifically, it's important to talk about what we want at the end of our life, and how we can vastly diminish the amount of energy and suffering that too often comes with trying to prolong life when nature calls. This is the purpose of an advance directive—a legal document you create to spell out your decisions about end-of-life care ahead of time. Our wishes are important to family, friends, and health-care professionals so there is no confusion down the road.

Hospitals generate seven times more revenue in patients who die within a year compared to those who live. "As a result, too many American deaths are still overly medicalized, robbing us of our chance at a peaceful passage," says internist Dr. John Schumann, also president of University of Oklahoma's Tulsa campus.

In some cases, it may be an individual's wish to de-medicalize death. Therefore, he/she should be prepared to express his/her care goals to die at home or in hospice.

One of the biggest problems that we face in not only modern society, but in now defunct societies as well, is that people have always been afraid to talk about death. In many cultures it is considered bad luck to talk about. I think to some extent that extends to this very day. Procuring a living will, having an advance directive, and, perhaps most importantly, having a designated health-care proxy, someone who can help transmit your decisions to a health-care team when you're not able to do so, is perhaps the most important thing that we can do for ourselves as patients and as human beings.

KEEP THE FAT BURNING FOR HEALTHY AGING

A number of factors are associated with aging gracefully that include virtually all the topics discussed throughout this book. Burning body fat by avoiding junk food and finding your optimal intake of natural carbohydrates is foremost, and as important, if not more, when we're seniors.

Keeping up with dietary changes to avoid becoming carbohydrate intolerant often leads many people into nutritional ketosis. In this case, you become less insulin resistant, and you achieve a more stable blood sugar level, a better hormone balance, a more functional brain, and many other health and fitness benefits, including a great metabolism.

The improved metabolism means we need fewer calories over the course of a typical day, which is a valuable benefit when aging.

For many people, this could be 10, 20, or even 30 percent fewer calories. This may be among the most powerful health benefits of reducing carbohydrate foods.

As we become better adapted to fat-burning, we can continue to maintain a highly efficient metabolism. As an example of our changing needs, one might require 2,000 calories at age fifty to maintain health and fitness, and at sixty, as carbohydrate intake needs to be reduced, we might now only require 1,600 calories a day, given the same amount of physical activity.

This can help biologically slow the aging process because it is associated with the reduction of oxidative (free radical) stress and improved immune function—something that we know occurs in humans when food intake is reduced and nutrients are not sacrificed.

KEEP THE BRAIN ENERGIZED!

Our little brain uses a disproportionate amount of energy for the size of our body. That's no surprise, considering all it has to do 24/7. But when that energy wanes, dysfunction develops, beginning years before the onset of memory loss, confusion, and other cognitive deficits. Much of this is preventable.

It's often said that the brain relies on glucose exclusively for energy. But this is not true. We would not have evolved without another fuel option, a backup so to speak. We have just the mechanism: the brain also can use ketone bodies for fuel very effectively to keep itself running well.

The aging brain may lose the ability to effectively rely on glucose as a primary fuel. When this happens, we begin to lose memory and other functions if we don't have a backup. In fact, Alzheimer's disease is associated with just this problem: the deterioration of the brain's ability to use glucose for energy. But it's not just Alzheimer's, as any loss of cognitive function can be associated with a "tired brain," one that is unable to rely on glucose for fuel to maintain high function. (The problem can exist in anyone and at any time throughout life, not just in the elderly.)

The reduction in the brain's use of glucose has been measured in studies long before brain symptoms first appear. Based on research by Stephen Cunnane and colleagues in a 2016 study in the *Annals of the New York Academy of Sciences*, the progression of brain dysfunction throughout life can often be described with this chart:

Early to mid-life	Aging	Later in life
No symptoms. Onset of poor glucose metabolism.	→ Deteriorating brain function. Onset of brain damage.	→ Symptoms of cognitive dysfunction. Brain cell death.

Enter our brain's backup energy source.

Ketones can keep our brains functioning very well. This can occur at any age, but is particularly important later in life when the brain loses some (or much) of its ability to use glucose. By consuming low-enough levels of carbohydrates with increased fat-burning, we can produce high levels of ketones to fuel the brain. As a general guide, this might be around 50 grams of carbohydrates a day, although as discussed throughout this book this level varies with the individual.

Among the many amazing clinical outcomes I've observed over my career has been with older individuals who, it was previously assumed, were experiencing permanent memory loss and other common cognitive deficits, only to find that when the brain is properly fueled with ketones, the person suddenly comes back to life.

THE FUTURE OF FAT-BURNING

Scientific support for low-carbohydrate and nutritional ketosis is finally gaining more credibility than ever, overcoming Big Sugar's grip on the world's major food supply. This became even more evident in my recent participation in the first-ever Conference on Nutritional Ketosis and Metabolic Therapeutics, in Tampa, Florida in January 2016. This refreshing and clinically hopeful look into the future of nutrition and fat-burning also brought to light the many challenges ahead.

It's now widely accepted that the ultimate fat-burning metabolic state is created by eating certain foods while avoiding others. As dietary carbohydrates are reduced and fats increased, the metabolism kicks in to burn more stored body fat for energy, both at rest and during physical activity. Excessive fatigue, pain, hunger, and many other abnormal signs and symptoms that can reduce quality of life can suddenly disappear. Many people, and clinicians, have known this for years, but suddenly the bandwagon is getting busier.

Nutritional ketosis can be applied as an approach to prevent and treat most of the common chronic diseases from Alzheimer's to cancer, and diabetes to heart disease. One of my earliest experiences with nutritional ketosis was a very successful two weeks of fasting when I was an undergraduate student. This involved only drinking water and eating no food. After a couple of days of feeling weak, I became energized from a high level of ketones, lost my hunger, and improved brain function. Fasting was also thought to be valuable in treating many chronic diseases, especially cancer.

Fast forward to today. We now know that fasting itself is not necessary to get the body to increase fat-burning and ketones significantly. You can do this simply by eating the right delicious foods.

The conference in Tampa was encouraging from the standpoint of the low-carb lifestyle and nutritional ketosis coming of age without any dramatic changes to the knowledge base formed over several decades; however, it also highlighted just how much work still needs to be done before this concept becomes accepted among the scientific community and general public.

Many of the studies presented, regarding the treatment of brain tumors and autism and resolutions regarding obesity and eliminating meds in diabetics, were published in mainstream medical journals. It was powerful data no one could ignore and everyone can use, if they choose. While the scientific stamp of approval has now been made, it must be noted that the scientific studies showing effectiveness are new and have yet to withstand the test of time.

Unfortunately, most practitioners will not suddenly recommend low-carbohydrate diets—unless, of course, one is drawn to it due to a personal health crisis. While small numbers of clinicians already recommend such eating habits, most still don't and won't make it a standard of care any time soon. Most still think it's crazy after all these years.

Ultimately the conference reinforced what some of us have been successfully applying for forty years—eating in a way that promotes the body's natural and powerful fat-burning metabolism leads to better health and human performance on all levels. And it's usually quite simple: Eat real food and find your level of natural carbohydrate needs to create the healthiest brain and body right now.

The future of fat-burning means that possibly, for the first time, populations can reduce the overfat pandemic. Whether this is actually accomplished is yet to be seen. One thing is certain—individuals who manage their health are most successful at eliminating excess body fat. It's all in your hands.

CHAPTER 11

A FEW OF MY FAVORITE FOODS

Just as "diets" can be unhealthy because people blindly follow them without consideration of whether those foods match our particular needs or not, recipes can do the same. Any cook-book approach is individualized. However, a great recipe means you have a great *idea* about how to make a delicious meal by adjusting it to your personal requirements. This chapter has some important ideas about creating quick, healthy meals and snacks, including travel food, that will help keep you from going off course in your journey to be a better fat-burner. You'll also find many recipes on my website: philmaffetone.com.

SOME BASICS

We live in a quick-food world, with fast-food drive-throughs and microwave meals. It has led to many people losing the ability to prepare meals from basic natural food ingredients.

In addition to choosing heathy, organic foods, how you prepare meals is important too. Consider these general guidelines:

- Meats, fish, and poultry can be oven- or pan-roasted, quickly grilled, and often cooked in their own juices. Fish is especially healthy when lightly steamed or poached and, when fresh and wild, can be eaten raw. Less oil or butter is needed for pan-cooking meats because they often contain their own fats. It's also important to avoid using high heat for too long. For instance, when grilling a steak or lamb, turn it every minute or so to prevent the excess formation of chemicals that can be harmful to your health. When grilling vegetables, turn them often as well. Ground meat should be bought fresh and cooked thoroughly as soon as possible. Many meat departments grind meat in the morning, so buy ground meats early in the day and cook or freeze them right away.
- The worst method for cooking is deep fat or high-heat frying using vegetable oils. Use monounsaturated and saturated fats for cooking, as they are not sensitive to heat. Coconut oil and butter are the safest fats for cooking, followed by olive oil, lard, and duck fat; the last three contain some polyunsaturated fats so care should be taken not to heat too high. Most other fats are high in polyunsaturated oils and very prone to oxidizing when exposed to heat, producing free radicals—avoid corn, safflower, sesame, soy, peanut, and canola oils.
- Vegetables can be steamed, stir-fried in olive oil, roasted, baked, or grilled. Cook vegetables minimally to avoid destroying nutrients; they also taste better when not

overcooked. If boiling or steaming, use as little water as possible to avoid the loss of nutrients through the water. Slow-cooked vegetable stews will contain much of the minerals and heat-resistant vitamins in the liquid while some heat-sensitive vitamins will be lost. Don't throw out the water from your steamed vegetables. Either drink it or use it for a soup base or in a smoothie.

- Eggs can be soft- or hard-boiled, cooked sunny-side up, over-easy, poached, or lightly scrambled. Letting the yolk remain soft is not only tastier but is healthier because heat-sensitive compounds are retained. Make sure the egg white cooks slightly because it's better for the intestines.

Buying and preparing the basics—meats, fish, eggs, cheese, vegetables, etc.—is often easy. Making them tasty is important too. This is accomplished quickly with some great dressings and sauces.

DRESSINGS AND SAUCES

The flavors of many foods can be heightened with a good dressing or sauce. Following are recipes for my favorite healthful salad dressings and stovetop sauces.

Phil's Salad Dressing

One of my first healthy habits, circa 1973, was creating this delicious dressing for many types of salads. It's simple: In a blender, mix 8 ounces extra virgin olive oil, 2 cloves garlic, 2 ounces or more apple cider vinegar, 1–2 tablespoons fresh or dried parsley (or cilantro), 1–2 teaspoons sea salt, and ½ teaspoon mustard.

Options:

- One to 2 tablespoons sheep or goat yogurt, or sour cream.
- Blend in 1 avocado, 1 tomato, 1 mango, or juice from half a lime (in place of the vinegar).
- Use 4 ounces of sesame, walnut, or avocado oil for variation in taste.

Once you find the best combinations, make a larger amount so you always have it available. Shake well before serving.

Spicy Sesame Ginger Dressing

Combine about 4 parts olive oil with 1 part rice wine vinegar. Add a small amount of sesame tahini, miso, grated ginger, salt, and chopped garlic.

Sauces make meals more exciting. Here are some simple ones.

Basic Butter Sauce

The most basic of sauces is also the easiest to make—simply butter and sea salt. After cooking vegetables, put some "sweet cream" butter on them while still hot, along with some sea salt. ("Sweet" butter is made without salt—the cream used to make this butter is a higher quality and tastier than that used for salted butter.) Even those who never liked vegetables will usually eat them with a butter sauce. Variation: sauté garlic or onions with or without some spices (tarragon works well) in butter.

Ghee or Clarified Butter

Melt one pound of sweet (unsalted) butter and bring just to the point of low boil to allow separation of solids and fat. Skim off solids that rise to the top (this can be added to soups or vegetables). Use the clear butter (ghee) like any other butter. Ghee does not burn like butter and does not require refrigeration.

Basic Tomato Sauce

This is a quick and easy, tasty, and healthful all-around red sauce. Just put some chopped fresh tomatoes or whole canned tomatoes in an uncovered pot and boil fast (not a simmer) until desired consistency. This may take a couple of hours or more, depending on the volume. Add salt. When cooked down to a thicker sauce, tomatoes take on a unique taste all their own. Even without adding any spices you'll have a great-tasting sauce. You can freeze it in small glass containers. Once you have the basic sauce, add garlic, parsley, basil, turmeric, or your favorite spices.

Basic Cream Sauce

The fanciest basic sauce is the cream sauce, simply made from heavy cream, butter, and salt. Use just less than the same amount of cream as the amount of sauce you want. For example, for about 2 cups of sauce, use a bit less than 2 cups of cream. Heat the cream to just before it simmers. Slowly add the hot cream to about a half-stick (4 tablespoons) of melted butter or ghee while continuously stirring over low to medium heat, bringing to a simmer for about five minutes (the longer you reduce it, the thicker it gets). For a thicker sauce, slowly stir in about ½ teaspoon finely ground psyllium. Add sea salt to taste.

Once you can make a good basic cream sauce, you can create a variety of different sauces almost as easily. For example, adding some chopped onion or garlic, a bay leaf, tarragon, or other spices to the cream, after heating it, makes a different sauce. For a cheese sauce, add any type of cheese to the basic cream sauce.

Sweet Basil Pesto

In a blender or food processor, mix fresh basil, garlic, extra virgin olive oil, pine nuts, and sea salt.

A DAY IN THE LIFE

Success in transitioning to healthy eating may depend, in part, on spending your natural carbohydrate "currency" wisely. This daily menu is an example, and has various sources of carbohydrates totaling 50 grams per day, which, for many people, results in nutritional ketosis. For some this level may not be necessary, while for others it could work very well. I don't normally recommend counting grams of foods, but below is an example of a full day's menu of 2,000 calories that includes 50 grams of carbohydrates. Adjust it to your own particular needs, whether raising or lowering the amount of food and calories, or adjusting the carbohydrate, protein, and fat content. This example is a very low-carbohydrate menu, with adequate protein and healthy fat.

Breakfast
Phil's Fat-Burning Organic Coffee (see recipe in chapter 4)
or
Eggs with sautéed zucchini in butter with fresh tomatoes

Lunch
Salad of mixed raw vegetables with half an avocado and 3 ounces raw or lightly cooked wild salmon in butter (or other meat)
Dressing: Extra virgin olive oil and balsamic vinegar

Mid-afternoon Smoothie
1–2 eggs
Raw vegetables (spinach, carrot)
1 tablespoon raw sesame seeds
½ small fresh apple

¼ cup blueberries
6 ounces water

Dinner
Cooked broccoli in butter and garlic
Duck (with skin) or beef steak
4 ounces red wine

Dessert
1½ ounces homemade Fast Fudge (recipe below)

Phil's Fast Fudge

- Melt 2 ounces of organic 100 percent pure cacao (sometimes called baking chocolate, without sugar) on warm temperature.
- Turn off heat and add 1 teaspoon honey, 1 tablespoon nut butter (cashew or almond) or tahini (sesame butter), and 1/8 teaspoon salt.
- Mix well and pour onto parchment paper or cups, or spread onto flat buttered plate to cool.
- Refrigerate.

Phil's basic Fast Fudge recipe is great, but here are some tasty ways to spice it up:

- Add ¼ teaspoon peppermint oil.
- Add 1 tablespoon of heavy cream to make it creamy.
- Almond or cashew butter center—premix very small amount of honey with the nut butter and place between thin layers of chocolate.
- Add unsweetened shredded coconut. Add about 2 tablespoons to dry mix before blending.
- Wrap a small piece of fudge around a whole roasted coffee bean.

Adjust honey to your particular needs.

HEALTHY SNACKS AND TRAVEL FOOD

Don't leave home without them!

While most snacks can add unhealthful and unwanted calories to your diet, this is only true if you eat the common junk food varieties. Healthful snacking can, in fact, help you control blood-sugar levels, improve metabolism, regulate stress, lower LDL cholesterol, burn more body fat, and increase energy levels. Snacking can keep hunger away, and reduce cravings for sugar.

Many people find that they have much more energy when following a program of healthy snacking. In addition, studies show a staggering 30 percent increase in heart disease in those eating three meals or fewer per day.

A key to smart snacking is to reduce the amount of food eaten at regular meals and distribute this nutritional wealth throughout the day. Skipping meals, in particular breakfast, may be one of the worst habits. Instead, eat five or six smaller meals that add up to the same amount of food that you would eat during your regular routine. This way, you're not adding more calories to your diet. Eating more frequently can increase fat-burning.

The easiest snack is leftovers of healthy meals you prepared earlier. Make a point of preparing more food, not only for snack but for another quick meal.

TRAVEL FOOD

One of the common problems with travel is finding nourishing food. The simple remedy for this is to bring your own. Whether you are spending the afternoon on the road, traveling by plane, or on a long train trip, you can bring along a diverse range of foods that are nutritional too.

Here are ten healthy travel foods; the first four can be consumed if you are taking the Two-Week Test:

- Raw almonds or cashews.
- Boiled eggs (peel and salt ahead of time, if desired).
- A small salad—quickly prepared and easily stored in a tight-fitting container. Adding cheese, eggs, and/or meat makes for a hearty meal. Don't forget the fork.
- The old standby—carrot and celery sticks. Add cucumbers, red peppers, and other veggies—and sea salt! These even go well with almond or cashew butter, or cream cheese.
- Fresh fruit. An organic apple won't squish in your pocket or carry-on, and makes an easy, nutritious snack. Add some full-fat cheese, and it becomes a travel meal.
- Plain unsweetened yogurt or sour cream with fresh fruit mixed in. It's quick to prepare in a jar or plastic container before leaving home. Don't forget the spoon.
- Another old standby—leftovers. Take some odds and ends from the previous day's meals and put them into one container.
- A smoothie in a tight-fitting container travels well too.

Real energy bars also make great travel food, and snacks. But buying them is a problem, as most are junk food. Instead, you can make your own.

PHIL'S BARS: FRESH, HEALTHY, AND ENERGIZING

For decades, one of my most popular creations has been the "Phil's Bar." The original came about through my desire to always have something healthy and convenient to eat while out and about, or unable to prepare a snack or meal. Over time there have been many different versions of Phil's Bars, as myself and others have adapted the recipe to suit our individual needs. But what has remained the same is they are fresh bars made from real food ingredients and are sweetened with just small amounts of honey. And they will last many days, even without refrigeration.

The traditional Phil's Bar is low-carb, and there is also a keto version for those eating very-low-carb.

Phil's Bar *Traditional*
Makes about 12 bars

3 cups raw almonds
⅔ cup egg white powder or whey concentrate powder
¼ cup cacao powder (also called pure unsweetened baker's chocolate)
⅓ cup honey
½ cup shredded coconut (unsweetened)

Nutrition Facts (approximations per bar, depending on size):
Calories 285
Carbohydrate 12g
Protein 12g
Fat 21g

Phil's Bar *Keto*
Makes about 12 bars

3 cups raw almonds
⅔ cup egg white powder or whey concentrate powder
¼ cup unsweetened baking chocolate (also called cacao paste)

¼ cup honey

½ cup shredded coconut (unsweetened)

Options: Add various healthy nuts such as pecans, macadamia, cashews, or combinations. In addition to vanilla, natural peppermint, almond, orange, or other oils can be used for added flavor.

Nutrition Facts (approximations per bar, depending on size):
Calories 300
Carbohydrate 10g
Protein 13g
Fat 23g

Instructions for both bars:

- Grind dry ingredients (a Cuisinart works best).
- In a separate bowl mix honey with an equal amount of hot water and vanilla, then blend into dry ingredients and mix well (you may have to mix it all by hand if your mixer isn't very efficient).
- If the batter is too wet, add a bit more dry ingredient; if too dry, add a bit more liquid.
- Adjust water/honey ratio for less or more sweetness.
- Shape into bars. You can also press the batter into a dish (about one-half to one-inch thick) and cut into bars. Or for fun shapes use a cookie cutter.
- They are best kept refrigerated but will typically last a week or more out of the refrigerator.

PLANT FOODS: TRY FOR TEN-A-DAY

Depending on your level of carbohydrate intolerance, healthy eating involves a balance of carbohydrates, proteins, and fats that matches your particular needs. This may include meat, fish, eggs, cheese, and a variety of natural fats such as olive oil, butter and ghee, coconut oil, lard, and others. Just as important are plant foods—vegetables and fruits as tolerated, along with nuts and seeds.

Trying for ten servings of plant foods is really not that unreasonable of a guideline, even though some sources recommend less. Long ago, our ancestors hunted primarily, and gathered when times were lean. It's even possible they consumed more plant food than they gathered by eating the contents of animal stomachs or other organs containing lots of vegetables and fruits.

While defining what's technically a vegetable or fruit is not precise, they are clearly plant foods. Typically, plant foods with a seed are fruits, but we tend to think of some less-sweet fruits like tomatoes and avocados as vegetables. Plants contain large amounts of nutrients. And if we are unable to eat a lot of fruit, other powerfully nutritious plant foods can be healthy too. Raw nuts and seeds are examples. The best are almonds, macadamia, pecans (the latter two lowest in carbs), with sesame being the better choice for seeds.

Making healthy plant foods a big part of each day means making them part of each meal or snack, including desserts. Here are some examples:

- Morning might include a hearty smoothie. Berries can complement spinach, and parsley, for example, along with raw sesame seeds.
- A vegetable omelet says it all, especially with a tomato sauce.
- Lunchtime salads with spinach, lettuce, avocado, and tomato is the foundation for a great meal when adding healthy-fat dressings and protein foods.

- A dinner of beef or fish could be complemented with a variety of vegetables cooked in butter or coconut oil with garlic, spices, or just salt.
- Healthy desserts can be berries and heavy (or whipped) cream.
- In the above day's scenario, it's easy to get ten servings of plant foods.

THE BEST NUTS AND SEEDS

The consumption of nuts and seeds has long been linked to reduced incidence of just about every major health problem, including cardiovascular disease, cancer, diabetes, and many others. One study linked a daily handful of nuts to a reduced risk of dying from any cause over a thirty-year period. Research shows that people who regularly eat nuts typically weigh less than those who don't. You do not necessarily need to eat large amounts to get benefits, either— small amounts regularly can improve your nutritional status.

Healthy nuts and seeds are typically low in carbohydrates (unless you eat too many), contain healthy amounts of fat, protein, and fiber, and are great sources of many vitamins and minerals.

The best nuts and seeds to eat are fresh, raw, and organic, and those with the best fat profiles. They should always be chewed well, or ground before using in recipes, to help digestion and allow for better absorption of the nutrients.

Nuts and seeds, like all foods, contain different ratios of certain fats. Those with higher levels of monounsaturated and lower levels of polyunsaturated fats are the most health-promoting. Roasting or otherwise cooking nuts and seeds, or leaving them unrefrigerated for long periods, can cause unhealthy oxidation of the polyunsaturated portion. This is evident if the taste is rancid or unnaturally bitter.

In fact, many nuts and seeds contain high levels of polyunsaturated fats, which is why these are not on the top-five list and should be consumed more sparingly. Some examples are the popular chia and traditional peanut (actually a legume), which are also lower in nutrients.

Nuts and seeds can be used to make delicious spreadable nut and seed butters, and can also be used in various healthy recipes, including smoothies, breads, pancakes/waffles, and desserts. As mentioned, cooking nuts and seeds can be harmful, so it's best to use those with lower polyunsaturated ratios, like almonds, cashews, and macadamias in recipes. Ground seeds are best used in recipes that will be consumed soon.

Based on these criteria, here are the five best nuts and seeds to consume regularly for better health:

- Almonds—The highest in monounsaturated fat, and low in polyunsaturated fat. They are good sources of protein and fiber, B2 and vitamin E, and the minerals magnesium and manganese.
- Cashews—Though they don't have quite the stellar fat ratios of almonds, tasty cashews also are relatively high in monounsaturated fat, and are a good source of protein. Cashews are not as high in vitamins and minerals, but do have more carbohydrates than almonds.
- Macadamia—Indigenous to Australia, with many grown in Hawaii, macadamia nuts are extremely high in monounsaturated fat and low in polyunsaturated fat. They are a very good source of vitamin B1 and the mineral manganese.
- Sesame—Sesame seeds contain good amounts of protein and fiber. Their fat profile is about half monounsaturated and half polyunsaturated so they should not be cooked. Buying unhulled seeds ensures fresh unspoiled healthy oils. They contain good amounts of various vitamins and minerals. Sesame seeds also contain the lignan *sesamin*, which is associated with several health benefits because of its natural anti-inflammatory effects.
- Flax—Many people view flax as an important source of omega-3 fat but the conversion to EPA (eicosapentaenoic acid), the important nutrient found in fish oil, is not very efficient and therefore flax is not a substitute for fish oil. However, these seeds are a good source of other nutrients, including B1, B6, and folate, as well as the minerals magnesium,

copper, and manganese. Flax is also rich in lignans and other phytonutrients. Always buy fresh whole flax seeds and consume them raw; soaking them or running them through a blender is OK and helps break down the hull to release nutrients. Like sesame, flax will become very unstable when broken or ground, so consume them soon.

Nuts are great additions to recipes like wheat-free bread, pancakes, waffles, and smoothies. A small handful can also make a great simple snack. Seeds are also great when ground for use in recipes that won't be cooked and will be consumed in a short period of time.

WHAT IS A SERVING?

The USDA defines a serving as one piece of fruit or a half cup of raw vegetables (except for greens, which is one cup of raw spinach, lettuce, kale, and others). Other dietary guidelines recommended different approaches for measuring servings. For instance, a serving of carrots might be one medium carrot; a serving of broccoli is one medium stalk; and a serving of asparagus is five spears.

Also consider dishes such as soups as a meal, which can easily include two or three servings of vegetables. Homemade tomato soup, for example, takes less than five minutes to prepare using fresh tomatoes.

I don't recommend juicing. Instead, by blending your vegetables, berries, and other plant foods whole, you'll get much more nutrition from the foods because you're not wasting the fiber and other nutrient-rich components that occurs with juicing.

Natural plant foods are a very important part of a healthy eating plan. They provide important vitamins, minerals, phytonutrients, and other nutrients essential for optimum health and fitness, and a key part of your plan to burn more body fat.

CHAPTER 12

CASE REPORTS

There are many experiences in the form of case reports I can present, but will limit the ones I describe here, since you now have the tools to make your own unique and successful case. Many readers will relate to the ones mentioned here. That's because the signs, symptoms, and scenarios are not that different when it comes to the common problem of carbohydrate intolerance, poor fat-burning, and the overfat condition. We now know that up to 76 percent of the world's adults and children are overfat, and in developed countries such as the US, the UK, Australia, and others, the numbers of overfat are shockingly into the high 80 percent range with children exceeding 50 percent.

By way of introducing this chapter, let's consider an example of a person who is born relatively healthy but falls into a long period of dysfunction with subtle but growing symptoms, ending with a diagnosis of disease. This case is a compilation of several real cases with a lot in common; so it's a hypothetical case report, but a valuable one to make here.

CASE REPORT 1

Some people begin life with undue stress. Our future patient may have been adversely affected by unhealthy food from the start, perhaps with formula rather than breastfeeding, or even sugar water shortly after birth. This type of stress could also have originated as maternal stress, as the mother's diet is shared by the baby for nine months. There could also be genetic factors, perhaps a diabetic grandparent, predisposing the baby to a less-stable blood-sugar mechanism, adversely affecting the brain. In this case, birth weight could be on the high or low range, and early development could demonstrate that the child is taller than most others in school.

During the early years of life, a number of unhealthy patterns and physiological imbalances may develop. By age ten, this carbohydrate-intolerant child may begin to develop symptoms that are perhaps associated with behavior or learning difficulties, hormonal issues, or even allergies or asthma. As time goes on, intestinal symptoms and fatigue may be more evident. Some experts have linked blood-sugar problems to drug use and criminal activity. For adolescents with such signs and symptoms, a pediatrician can usually rule out more clearly defined problems or disease, but usually the conclusion is that the symptoms may just be part of growing.

Before reaching age twenty, this person is probably overfat. Attempts to lose weight, if any, come through dieting. This usually vacillates from starving his or herself to lowering fat intake, accompanied by increased consumption of carbohydrates. It can also begin the process of yo-yo dieting, in which a lower caloric intake decreases metabolism, which sometimes results in some short-term weight loss, with the final consequence of weight gain. There is now an eating disorder, in some cases on the mild side of the spectrum. Body fat worsens.

Up to this point, this person would probably not have sought traditional health care for these seemingly minor but annoying problems. Over-the-counter drugs and other remedies such as increasing reliance on caffeine and energy drinks for fueling provide symptomatic relief, but the cause is never sought or found.

For those in their twenties and thirties, the carbohydrate-intolerant person usually becomes a patient, choosing a specialty based on the most uncomfortable symptoms, or finding a primary care practitioner. Many of the symptoms have now worsened: fatigue, intestinal bloating, and decreased concentration. Pain occurs too easily now. Addictions are common—sometimes to sweets, caffeine, alcohol, tobacco, or over-the-counter or illicit drugs. Medication is commonly prescribed.

Many symptoms are now easily observed and measurable by a practitioner. Dizziness, caused by a significant blood-pressure drop upon standing, is common. Blood pressure may begin to elevate, enough for the patient to be diagnosed with pre-hypertension. Abnormal glucose-tolerance tests are sometimes found, but more often fasting blood sugar is within normal limits. Sleep may be disturbed. Other signs include increased belly fat. Blood fats, especially triglycerides but also cholesterol, may begin to increase above acceptable limits.

The patient may be put on a medically supervised "diet" to help reduce weight. This would usually be high in carbohydrates, and low in fat, red meat, eggs, and cheese. The symptoms, and the overfat state, might just get worse.

Exercise is sometimes recommended too. But with no individualization, the patient may exercise too intensely in the hope of burning more calories. This leads to further reduced fat-burning.

As the patient climbs toward feeling "over-the-hill" at age forty, health continues to worsen. Now with hypertension and high LDL cholesterol and triglycerides, a slightly elevated blood sugar level leads to a diagnosis of prediabetes. The risk for heart disease is now very high. Lifestyle changes, which were not taken seriously before, are now not considered as the patient's health has deteriorated too much.

This patient's so-called golden years can literally be quite difficult for both patient and family, and a great expense for all, including society. Our patient, now a medicated, hypertensive, overfat diabetic on the verge of requiring bypass surgery, remains at high risk until the end. But modern medicine has helped lengthen the life span. When death comes, it comes with pain and suffering.

Could this scenario be changed? Clearly the answer is yes. And it's not just a philosophy, it's real. But we can't go back and change it; now is the time to do so.

CASE REPORT 2

JB came to my clinic with a dilemma, having worked out regularly, while keeping calories in check for over a year. Yet, body fat would not budge, muscles felt weak, and mental and physical energy levels were low. After an extensive physical evaluation and dietary analysis, the remedy seemed simple: slow down, avoid junk food, stay off the scale, and eat healthy fats. JB was game. Within two weeks, JB felt like a new person. Long-standing hunger was gone, food was enjoyable again, and workouts were fun and exhilarating. Within a month, friends were asking whether weight was reduced. "Don't know, I'm not supposed to get on the scale," JB said—a comment that brought some strange looks. But when clothes clearly began fitting more loosely, JB just had to take a peek at the scale—no weight loss! Having called my clinic in a panic, JB asked for an explanation. I explained how the loss of body fat resulted in leanness: Because more body fat was being burned—resulting in increased energy—both fatigue and hunger dissolved. While workouts seemed easy, muscles strengthened. The combination of a slight increase in muscle, whose mass added a few pounds of weight, and body fat loss, which doesn't weigh much but takes up more space, caused the scale weight to even out. JB finally understood what was going on, happily declaring, "It's about time."

CASE REPORT 3

While few clinicians and coaches recommend low-carbohydrate/high-fat eating plans to improve athletic performance, recent published studies have demonstrated their value. Potential benefits include improved training and racing energy through increased fat-burning, reductions in caloric requirements (food intake) during training and competition, and the reduced incidence of serious gastrointestinal complaints common in competitive endurance athletes. RP is a 38-year-old professional triathlete of 13 years who began reducing carbohydrate foods while increasing fat intake in an attempt to improve a number of serious health problems, and improve race performance. The health problems included serious, chronic gastrointestinal problems, fatigue, and significant hormone imbalance that caused debilitating menstrual signs and symptoms. Over the course of six weeks, beginning with the Two-Week Test, RP reduced her carbohydrate content from 73 percent to 12 percent, fat content increased from 14 percent to 75 percent, and protein levels remained constant at 13 percent. Training intensity was reduced to further help improve fat-burning. Waist size and physical energy improved.

Between May and November, three Ironman events were successfully completed. Pre-race meals were now high-fat instead of high-carb: approximately 20g carbohydrates, 20g protein, and 100g fat (total 1060 kcal). Compared to previous years, race calories consumed were reduced from 400 per hour to 130 per hour. All gastrointestinal and hormone signs and symptoms disappeared. Two races were personal best times, with the final Ironman Triathlon completed in an amazing 8 hours 52 minutes.

CASE REPORT 4

Bob was determined to renew his health in a natural way. Despite being normal weight, he was clearly overfat, always exhausted, and his blood pressure, cholesterol, and triglycerides were alarmingly high. He started the Two-Week Test and initially felt very good. But within a few days he began getting tired and irritable. After talking with Bob on the phone for just a few minutes, it was clear that he was doing several things wrong. By calculating how many calories he was eating, Bob became calorie-conscious and purposely ate less fat. To make matters worse, he thought that yogurt was in the cheese group, and was eating two to three containers of fruit yogurt each day. When I told Bob that the yogurt he was eating had 6 to 7 teaspoons of sugar in each container, and to forget about the calories for now, he started his test again. After the first week he was feeling much better. Within a month, his energy remained high, and a couple of months after that, his visit to his primary doctor showed his blood pressure and blood fats were back to normal, and he had lost 14 pounds and had to buy new clothes.

CASE REPORT 5

Sally's history was not unusual. At age thirty, she decided to get serious about taking off the excess weight she accumulated over the past decade. So she followed a low-calorie diet that limited her intake to 1,000 calories per day. Within three months, Sally felt more tired and ravenous, but finally reached her goal of losing 20 pounds. Six months later, she gained about 25 pounds back. She returned to her diet, and it was just as successful as before, although it took a little longer to lose the 25 pounds. This vicious cycle continued for about five years. Sally was now not only tired, but also depressed, and had insomnia and PMS for two weeks each month. During my initial consultation with Sally, I explained how she continually impaired her fat-burning, and her metabolism was getting worse with each vicious cycle. Sally was weaned off her calorie-counting and eventually was able to eat as much as her body required without hunger. In time she got down to the same size clothes she wore when she was at her "ideal" weight at twenty-two years of age. And to her surprise, she was eating about 2,000 calories each day.

CASE REPORT 6

SR was very dedicated to her exercise routine. She went to aerobic dance class four mornings a week, and walked twice weekly with friends. But her time was not well spent, she thought, since body fat was not changing much in the two years she worked out. She also was very tired on the days she did aerobics. I asked SR to wear a heart monitor during her aerobics class and when she walked. Not surprisingly, her heart rate exceeded 180 beats per minute during aerobics, and averaged 155 on her walks. I determined that SR's aerobic heart rate for optimal fat-burning was 140. Thus she had programmed her body to burn more sugar and less fat. After seeing that she couldn't physically perform the aerobic routine during an advanced class without her heart rate easily going over 140, SR went to an easier class where she was able to control her heart rate at 140. She also began walking on her own, at a much slower pace. Within a couple of months, SR lost more weight than in the previous two years, her workouts now gave her energy, and she became much leaner. In time, she was able to go back to the advanced aerobics class and walk with her friends while maintaining a 140 heart rate.

CASE REPORT 7

Dave, a former college all-American, was in his mid-forties, overweight, and feeling the effects of work stress. Since he was in the athletic apparel business, he wanted to appear more fit. He began walking on the high school track almost every evening. He got out of breath and tired easily, so he kept his pace relatively slow. After a couple of months with virtually no results, Dave asked for help. I told him to perform his walk as he usually does, but with a heart monitor. To our surprise, his heart rate exceeded 170 and stayed there for nearly the entire workout. Once Dave began using a heart monitor regularly and kept his rate at the prescribed level of 130 beats per minute by walking even more slowly, it was only a couple of weeks before he felt some positive results. And within a couple of months, Dave was thinner, had more energy, and was walking faster at the same heart rate.

CASE REPORT 8

For more than five hours of rigorous racing in the Colorado Rockies, Hal relied on water only, and his stored body fat for fuel.

Hal won the 29-mile World Championship Pack Burro Race for the seventh time, running with a jenny named Full Tilt Boogie, and using training and nutrition methods he's learned by being one of my editors over the past twenty years.

This annual event is held on a rugged mountainous course from the town of Fairplay, elevation 10,000 feet, to the top of 13,187-foot Mosquito Pass, and back to Fairplay. Competitors run and hike the steeper pitches with their burros but may not ride. The animals carry 33-pound packs, including a pick, pan, and shovel to commemorate the state's mining history.

Hal says the race is much more demanding than a typical marathon or triathlon due to the extremes in elevation, vertical gain, weather conditions, and terrain, not to mention managing an animal not known for its cooperative nature. He's also competed in marathons, ultramarathons, and winter multi-sport competitions.

Hal attributes his success to a high degree of fat-burning achieved over the years of training using aerobic training and a diet customized to suit his needs. He notes that he drank only water and ate nothing during the entire event, an indication of an excellent fat-burning capacity.

Hal also notes he does very little anaerobic training, but this did not keep him from having a finishing kick.

The race boiled down to a contest between Hal and another team, who traded places as many as thirty times over the course of the event, with Hal and Boogie finally pulling ahead near the finish line, winning in 5 hours, 25 minutes and 23 seconds, two seconds ahead of the second-place team.

This was Hal's seventh world championship in fifteen years and, at age fifty-three, it is believed he is the oldest person to win in the sixty-five-year history of the event.

CONCLUSION

There is one case report missing in the previous chapter: yours. It's the most important one that only you can create. Whether you keep it personal or shout it out to the world is up to you. Nothing makes me feel better than to see others take this information and truly run with it, especially when sharing it to influence others in their own personal journey to better health and fitness.

There may appear to be a lot of information in this book, especially if it's new to you and even if much of it is quite different from what you used to think. Implementing it, though, is really quite simple. Eat real food and avoid junk.

In coming this far in your reading, congratulations on taking that all-important first big step. A key part of this step is deciding you're going to better manage your health, in particular be a better fat burner to help reduce unhealthy excess body fat.

In managing the process, sometimes with the help of one or more like-minded health practitioners, you'll no doubt want to return to some topics in the book to better understand the process. If you want more information, it can be found in my *Big Book of Health and Fitness*. If you're a competitive athlete, my *Big Book of Endurance Training and Racing* will also describe how to reach your athletic potential. For everyone, my website provides the latest articles and updates: www.philmaffetone.com.

The idea that a healthy brain can help guide our personal food choices is quite real and natural, at least once we escape sugar addiction, or even just reduce carbohydrate intolerance so our intuition better guides us. This is a goal of the Two-Week Test, another key step, with the third important one determining your personal level of natural carbohydrate intake.

For more than forty years I have been fortunate enough to help people successfully apply the notion that eating in a way that promotes the body's natural and powerful fat-burning metabolism leads to better health and human performance on all levels. Equipped with this knowledge, you are now in control.

ENDNOTES

1. Marlene B. Schwartz, Lenny R. Vartanian, Brian A. Nosek, and Kelly D. Brownell, "The Influence of One's Own Body Weight on Implicit and Explicit Anti-fat Bias," *Obesity* 14 (2006): 440–447.
2. Philip B. Maffetone, Ivan Rivera-Dominguez, and Paul B. Laursen, "Overfat and Underfat: New Terms and Definitions Long Overdue," *Front Public Health* ," 4 (2017): 279.

BIBLIOGRAPHY

Affenito SG, Backstrand JR, Welch GW, Lammi-Keefe CJ, Rodriguez NR, Adams CH. Subclinical and clinical eating disorders in IDDM negatively affect metabolic control. Diabetes Care. 1997; 20(2): 182–184.

Ali S, Garcia JM. Sarcopenia, cachexia, and aging: diagnosis, mechanisms, and therapeutic options. Gerontology. 2014; 60(4): 294–305.

Alwan A, Armstrong T, Bettcher D, et al. Global status report on noncommunicable diseases 2010. Geneva: World Health Organization; 2011.

Andersen C, Clarsen B, Johansen T, Engebretsen L. High prevalence of overuse injury among iron-distance triath-letes. Br J Sports Med. 2013; 47(13): 857–861.

Anker SD, von Haehling S. Cachexia as a major underes-timated and unmet medical need: facts and numbers. J Cachexia Sarcopenia Muscle. 2010; 1(1): 1–5.

Aspen V, Weisman H, Vannucci A, et al. Psychiatric co-mor-bidity in women presenting across the continuum of dis-ordered eating. Eat Behav. 2014; 15(4): 686–693.

Atlantis E, Martin SA, Haren MT, AW Taylor, GA Wittert, Members of the Florey Adelaide Male Ageing Study. Inverse associations between muscle mass, strength, and the metabolic syndrome. Metabolism. 2009; 58: 1013–1022.

Bartlett JD, Louhelainen J, Iqbal Z, et al. Reduced carbohydrate availability enhances exercise-induced p53 signaling in human skeletal muscle: implications for mitochondrial biogenesis. Am J Physiol Regul Integr Comp Physiol. 2013; 304(6): R450-R458.

Baumgartner RN, Heymsfield SB, Roche AF. Human body composition and the epidemiology of chronic disease. Obesity Research. 1995; 3(1): 73–95.

Bazzano LA, Hu T, Reynolds K, et al. Effects of low-carbohydrate and low-fat diets: a randomized trial. Ann Intern Med. 2014; 161(5): 309–318.

Bloom DE, Cafiero ET, Jané-Llopis E, et al. The global economic burden of noncommunicable diseases. Geneva: World Economic Forum; 2011.

Bonci CM, Bonci LJ, Granger LR, et al. National athletic trainers' association position statement: preventing, detecting, and managing disordered eating in athletes. J Athl Train. 2008; 43(1): 80–108.

Bray GA. Contemporary diagnosis and management of obesity and the metabolic syndrome. Newtown, PA: Handbooks in Health Care; 2003.

Brehm BJ, Seeley RJ, Daniels SR, D'Alessio DA. A randomized trial comparing a very low carbohydrate diet and a calorie-restricted low fat diet on body weight and cardiovascular risk factors in healthy women. J Clin Endocrinol Metab. 2003; 88: 1617–1623.

Brinkworth GD, Noakes M, Buckley JD, Keogh JB, Clifton PM. Long-term effects of a very-low-carbohydrate weight loss diet compared with an isocaloric low-fat diet after 12 mo. Am J Clin Nutr. 2009; 90: 23–32.

Bruera E, Strasser F, Palmer JL, et al. Effect of fish oil on appetite and other symptoms in patients with advanced cancer and anorexia/cachexia: a double-blind, placebo-controlled study. J Clin Oncol. 2003; 21(1): 129–134.

Buchheit M, Simpson BM, Schmidt WF, et al. Predicting sickness during a 2-week soccer camp at 3600 m (ISA3600). Br J Sports Med. 2013; 47 Suppl 1: i124-i127.

Cavicchia PP, Steck SE, Hurley TG, et al. A new dietary inflammatory index predicts interval changes in serum high-sensitivity C-reactive protein. J Nutr. 2009; 139(12): 2365–2372.

Centers for Disease Control and Prevention (CDC). Trends in intake of energy and macronutrients—United States, 1971–2000. MMWR Morb Mortal Wkly Rep. 2004; 53(4): 80–82.

Centers for Disease Control and Prevention (CDC). Adult participation in aerobic and muscle-strengthening physical activities—United States, 2011. MMWR Morb Mortal Wkly Rep. 2013; 62(17): 326–330.

Coussens LM, Werb Z. Inflammation and cancer. Nature Rev Immunol. 2002; 420(6917): 860–867.

Dagan SS, Segev S, Novikov I, Dankner R. Waist circumference vs body mass index in association with cardiorespiratory fitness in healthy men and women: a cross sectional analysis of 403 subjects. Nutr J. 2013; 12(1): 12.

DePalma MT. Identifying college athletes at risk for pathogenic eating. Br J Sports Med. 2002; 36: 45–50.

Deurenberg P, Yap M, van Staveren WA. Body mass index and percent body fat: a meta analysis among different ethnic groups. Int J Obes Relat Metab Disord. 1998; 22: 1164–1171.

Donath MY, Shoelson SE. Type 2 diabetes as an inflammatory disease. Nat Rev Immun. 2011; 11(2): 98–107.

Ellis AC, Hyatt TC, Gower BA, Hunter GR. Respiratory quotient predicts fat mass gain in premenopausal women. Obesity (Silver Spring). 2010; 18(12): 2255–2259.

Esteve-Lanao J, Foster C, Seiler S, Lucia A. Impact of training intensity distribution on performance in endurance athletes. J Strength Cond Res. 2007; 21(3): 943–949.

Farkas J, von Haehling S, Kalantar-Zadeh K, Morley JE, Anker SD, Lainscak M. Cachexia as a major public health problem: frequent, costly, and deadly. J Cachexia Sarcopenia Muscle. 2013; 4(3): 173–178.

Faulkner JA. Terminology for contractions of muscles during shortening, while isometric, and during lengthening. J App Physio. 2003; 95(2): 455–459.

Feinman RD, Pogozelski WK, Astrup A, et al. Dietary carbohydrate restriction as the first approach in diabetes management: critical review and evidence base. Nutrition. 2015; 31(1): 1–13.

Festa A, D'Agostino R Jr, Williams K, et al. The relation of body fat mass and distribution to markers of chronic inflammation. Int J Obes Relat Metab Disord. 2001; 25(10): 1407–1415.

Foster GD, Wyatt HR, Hill JO, et al. Weight and metabolic outcomes after 2 years on a low-carbohydrate versus low-fat diet: a randomized trial. Ann Intern Med. 2010; 153:(3) 147–157.

Freedman DS, Ford ES. Are the recent secular increases in the waist circumference of adults independent of changes in BMI? Am J Clin Nutr. 2015; 101(3): 425–431.

Frellick M. Obesity now more common than underweight worldwide. Medscape Medical News; 2016 (http://www.medscape.com/viewarticle/861383).

Gaida JE, Alfredson H, Kiss ZS, Bass SL, Cook JL. Asymptomatic Achilles tendon pathology is associated with a central fat distribution in men and a peripheral fat distribution in women: a cross sectional study of 298 individuals. BMC Musculoskelet Disord. 2010; 11: 41.

Gallagher D, Heymsfield SB, Heo M, Jebb SA, Murgatroyd PR, Sakamoto Y. Healthy percentage body fat ranges: an approach for developing guidelines based on body mass index. Am J Clin Nutr. 2000; 72(3): 694–701.

Gibala MJ, McGee SL. Metabolic adaptations to short-term high-intensity interval training: a little pain for a lot of gain? Exerc Sport Sci Rev. 2008; 36(2): 58–63.

Gonzalez MJ, Miranda-Massari JR. Diet and stress. Psychiatr Clin North Am. 2014; 37(4): 579–589.

Hak PT, Hodzovic E, Hickey B. The nature and prevalence of injury during CrossFit training. J Strength Cond Res. 2013. doi: 10.1519/JSC.0000000000000318.

Harber MP, Gallagher PM, Creer AR, Minchev KM, Trappe SW. Single muscle fiber contractile properties during a competitive season in male runners. Am J Physiol Regul Integr Comp Physiol. 2004; 287(5): R1124-R1131.

Hetlelid KJ, Plews DJ, Herold E, Laursen PB, Seiler S. Rethinking the role of fat oxidation: substrate utilisation during high-intensity interval training in well-trained and recreationally trained runners. BMJ Open Sport Exerc Med. 2015; 1(1): e000047.

Heymsfield SB, Ebbeling CB, Zheng J, et al. Multi-component molecular level body composition reference methods:

evolving concepts and future directions. Obes Rev. 2015; 16(4): 282–94.

Hind K, Gannon L, Brightmore A, Beck B. Insights into relationships between body mass, composition and bone: findings in elite rugby players. J Clin Densitom. 2015; 18(2): 172–178.

Høeg T, Maffetone P. The development and initial assessment of a novel heart rate training formula. Poster presented at the Medicine & Science in Ultra-Endurance Sports 2nd Annual Conference; May 2015; Olympic Valley, CA, USA.

Hu T, Mills KT, Yao L, et al. Effects of low-carbohydrate diets versus low-fat diets on metabolic risk factors: A meta-analysis of randomized controlled clinical trials. Am J Epidemiol. 2012; 176(Suppl7): S44–S54.

Hunma S, Ramuth H, Miles-Chan JL, et al. Body composition-derived BMI cut-offs for overweight and obesity in Indians and Creoles of Mauritius: comparison with Caucasians. Inter J Obesity. 2016; 40(12): 1906–1914.

Hutley L, Prins JB. Fat as an endocrine organ: relationship to the metabolic syndrome. Am J Med Sci. 2005; 330(6): 2548–2556.

Jiang SZ, Lu W, Zong XF, Ruan HY, Liu Y. Obesity and hypertension. Exp Ther Med. 2016; 12(4): 2395–2399.

Kershaw EE, Flier JS. Adipose tissue as an endocrine organ. J Clin Endocrin Metab. 2004; 89(6): 2548–2556.

Kim J, Peterson KE, Scanlon KS, et al. Trends in overweight from 1980 through 2001 among preschool-aged children enrolled in a health maintenance organization. Obesity (Silver Spring). 2006; 14(7): 1107–1112.

Koenig W, Sund M, Fröhlich M, et al. C-reactive protein, a sensitive marker of inflammation, predicts future risk of coronary heart disease in initially healthy middle-aged men results from the MONICA (Monitoring Trends and Determinants in Cardiovascular Disease) Augsburg Cohort Study, 1984 to 1992. Circulation. 1999; 99(2): 237–242.

Koh-Banerjee P, Wang Y, Hu FB, Spiegelman D, Willett WC, Rimm EB. Changes in body weight and body fat distribution as risk factors for clinical diabetes in US men. Am J Epidemiol. 2004; 159(12): 1150–1159.

Kreher JB, Schwartz JB. Overtraining syndrome: a practical guide. Sports Health. 2012; 4(2): 128–138.

Lee J, Lee JY, Lee JH, et al. Visceral fat obesity is highly associated with primary gout in a metabolically obese but normal weighted population: a case control study. Arthritis Res Ther. 2015; 17(1): 79.

Lee IM, Shiroma EJ, Lobelo F, et al. Effect of physical inactivity on major non-communicable diseases worldwide: an analysis of burden of disease and life expectancy. Lancet. 2012; 380(9838): 219–229.

Leroy L, Bayliss E, Domino M, et al. The Agency for Healthcare Research and Quality Multiple Chronic Conditions Research Network: Overview of research contributions and future priorities. Med Care. 2014; 52 (Suppl 3): S15-S22.

Li C, Ford ES, Zhao G, Balluz LS, Giles WH. Estimates of body composition with dual-energy X-ray absorptiometry in adults. Am J Clin Nutr. 2009; 90(6): 1457–1465.

Lindsberg PJ, Grau AJ. Inflammation and infections as risk factors for ischemic stroke. Stroke. 2003; 34(10): 2518–2532.

Lobstein T, Baur L, Uauy R, IASO International Obesity TaskForce. Obesity in children and young people: a crisis in public health. Obesity Rev. 2004; 5(Suppl 1): 4–104.

Loucks AB, Redman LM. The effect of stress on menstrual function. Trends Endocrinol Met. 2004; 15(10): 466–471.

Maffetone P. Complementary sports medicine. Champaign, IL: Hum Kinet; 1999.

Maffetone P, Laursen PB. Athletes: Fit but unhealthy? Sports Med Open. 2016; 2(1): 24.

Maffetone P, Laursen PB. Case study: Reductions in training load and dietary carbohydrates help restore health and improve performance in an Ironman triathlete. Int J Sports Sci Coaching. July 2017. In press.

Mantovani G, Madeddu C, Macciò A, et al. Cancer-related anorexia/cachexia syndrome and oxidative stress: an innovative approach beyond current treatment. Cancer Epidemiol Biomark Prev. 2004; 13(10): 1651–1659.

Marquet LA, Brisswalter J, Louis J, et al. Enhanced endurance performance by periodization of carbohydrate intake: "sleep low" strategy. Med Sci Sports Exerc. 2016; 48(4): 663–672.

Martin AB, Hartman M, Benson J, Catlin A, National Health Expenditure Accounts Team. National health spending in 2014: faster growth driven by coverage expansion and prescription drug spending. Health Affairs. 2016; 35(1): 150–160.

Martinsen M, Sundgot-Borgen J. Higher prevalence of eating disorders among adolescent elite athletes than controls. Med Sci Sports Exer. 2013; 45(6): 1188–1197.

Mattson MP, Allison DB, Fontana L, et al. Meal frequency and timing in health and disease. Proc Natl Acad Sci USA. 2014; 111(47): 16647–16653.

Melton LJ 3rd, Khosla S, Crowson CS, O'Connor MK, O'Fallon WM, Riggs BL. Epidemiology of sarcopenia. J Am Geriatr Soc. 2000; 48(6): 625–630.

Menke A, Casagrande S, Geiss L, Cowie C. Prevalence of and trends in diabetes among adults in the United States, 1988–2012. JAMA. 2015; 314(10): 1021–1029.

Misra A, Anoop S, Gulati S, Mani Ka, Bhatt SP, Pandey RM. Body fat patterning, hepatic fat and pancreatic volume of non-obese Asian Indians with type 2 diabetes in North India: a case control study. PLoS One. 2015; 10(10): e0140477.

Morley JE, Thomas DR, Wilson MM. Cachexia: pathophysiology and clinical relevance. Am J Clin Nutr. 2006; 83(4): 735–743.

Morris MJ, Beilharz JE, Maniam J, Reichelt AC, Westbrook RF. Why is obesity such a problem in the 21st century? The intersection of palatable food, cues and reward pathways, stress, and cognition. Neurosci Biobehav Rev. 2015; 58: 36–45.

Mumford SL, Chavarro JE, Zhang C, et al. Dietary fat intake and reproductive hormone concentrations and ovulation in regularly menstruating women. Am J Clin Nutr. 2016; 103(3): 868–877.

Munoz I, Seiler S, Alcocer A, Carr N, Esteve-Lanao J. Specific intensity for peaking: is race pace the best option? Asian J Sports Med. 2015; 6(3): e24900. doi: 10.5812/asjsm.24900.

National Eating Disorders Collaboration. NEDC e-Bulletin, Issue 19, February 2014 (http://www.nedc.com.au/files/enews/NEDC%20e-Bulletin%20February%202014.pdf).

National Institute on Aging, National Institutes of Health. Why population aging matters: A global perspective. Bethesda, MD: National Institute on Aging; 2007.

National Institutes of Health. The practical guide to the identification, evaluation, and treatment of overweight and obesity in adults. Bethesda, MD: National Institutes of Health; 2000.

NCD Risk Factor Collaboration (NCD-RisC). Trends in adult body-mass index in 200 countries from 1975 to 2014: a pooled analysis of 1698 population-based measurement studies with 19.2 million participants. Lancet. 2016; 387(10026): 1377–1396.

Ng M, Fleming T, Robinson M, et al. Global, regional, and national prevalence of overweight and obesity in children and adults during 1980–2013: a systematic analysis for the Global Burden of Disease Study 2013. Lancet. 2014; 384(9945): 766–781.

Noakes T, Volek JS, Phinney SD. Low-carbohydrate diets for athletes: what evidence? Br J Sports Med. 2014; 48(14): 1077–1078.

Noakes TD. Low-carbohydrate and high-fat intake can manage obesity and associated conditions: occasional survey. S Afr Med J. 2013; 103(11): 826–830.

O'Connor DB, Armitage CJ, Ferguson E. Randomized test of an implementation intention-based tool to reduce stress-induced eating. Ann Behav Med. 2015; 49(3): 331–343.

Ogden CL, Carroll MD, Curtin LR, McDowell MA, Tabak CJ, Flegal KM. Prevalence of overweight and obesity in the United States, 1999–2004. JAMA. 2006; 295(13): 1549–1555.

Oliver CJ. Not being able to see the muscle for the fat. J Cachexia Sarcopenia Muscle. 2012; 3(1): 69–70.

Oliveros E, Somers VK, Sochor O, Goel K, Lopez-Jimenez F. The concept of normal weight obesity. Prog Cardiovasc Dis. 2014; 56(4): 426–433.

Patry-Parisien J, Shields M, Bryan S. Comparison of waist circumference using the World Health Organization and National Institutes of Health protocols. Statistics Canada, Catalogue no. 82-003-XPE. Health Reports, Vol. 23, no. 3, September 2012. (http://www.statcan.gc.ca/pub/82-003-x/2012003/article/11707-eng.htm).

Phinney SD, Bistrian BR, Evans WJ, Gervino E, Blackburn GL. The human metabolic response to chronic ketosis without caloric restriction: preservation of submaximal exercise capability with reduced carbohydrate oxidation. Metabolism. 1983; 32(8): 769–776.

Pokharel Y, Basra S, Lincoln AE, et al. Association of body mass index and waist circumference with subclinical atherosclerosis in retired NFL players. Southern Med J. 2014; 107(10): 633–639.

Pradhan AD, Manson JE, Rifai N, Buring JE, Ridker PM. C-reactive protein, interleukin 6, and risk of developing type 2 diabetes mellitus. JAMA. 2001; 286(3): 327–334.

Prospective Studies Collaboration, Whitlock G, Lewington S, et al. Body-mass index and cause-specific mortality in 900,000 adults: collaborative analyses of 57 prospective studies. Lancet. 2009; 373(9669): 1083–1096.

Renfrew Center Foundation for Eating Disorders. Eating disorders 101 guide: A summary of issues, statistics and resources. Renfrew Center Foundation for Eating Disorders, 2002 Sept, revised 2003 Oct.

Riedl A, Vogt S, Holle R, et al. Comparison of different measures of obesity in their association with health-related quality of life in older adults - results from the KORA-Age study. Public Health Nutr. 2016; 19(18): 3276–3286.

Ruderman N, Chisholm D, Pi-Sunyer X, Schneider S. The metabolically obese, normal-weight individual revisited. Diabetes. 1998; 47(5): 699–713.

Ruderman NB, Berchtold P, Schneider S. Obesity associated disorders in normal-weight individuals: some speculations. Int J Obes. 1982; 6 Suppl 1: 151–157.

Ruderman NB, Schneider SH, Berchtold P. The "metaboli-cally-obese," normal-weight individual. Am J Clin Nutr. 1981; 34(8): 1617–1621.

Ruiz JR, Sui X, Lobelo F, et al. Association between muscular strength and mortality in men: prospective cohort study. BMJ. 2008; 337: a439.

Sakuma K, Yamaguchi A. Sarcopenic obesity and endocrinal adaptation with age. Int J Endocrinol. 2013; 2013: 204164. doi: 10.1155/2013/204164.

Sav A, McMillan SS, Kelly F, et al. The ideal healthcare: pri-orities of people with chronic conditions and their carers. BMC Health Serv Res. 2015; 15:551.

Schmitt L, Regnard J, Millet GP. Monitoring fatigue status with HRV measures in elite athletes: an avenue beyond RMSSD? Front Physiol. 2015; 6: 343.

Scott IA, Hilmer SN, Reeve E, et al. Reducing inappropriate polypharmacy: the process of deprescribing. JAMA Intern Med. 2015; 175(5): 827–834.

Shai I, Schwarzfuchs D, Henkin Y, et al. Weight loss with a low-carbohydrate, Mediterranean, or low-fat diet. N Engl J Med. 2008; 359(3): 229–241.

Shen W, Punyanitya M, Chen J, et al. Waist circumference correlates with metabolic syndrome indicators better than percentage fat. Obesity (Silver Spring). 2006; 14(4): 727–736.

Shingleton RM, Richards LK, Thompson-Brenner H. Using technology within the treatment of eating disorders: a clinical practice review. Psychotherapy (Chic). 2013; 50(4): 576–582.

Smalley KJ, Knerr AN, Kendrick ZV, Colliver JA, Owen OE. Reassessment of body mass indices. Am J Clin Nut. 1990; 52(3): 405–8.

Srikanthan P, Karlamangla AS. Relative muscle mass is inversely associated with insulin resistance and pre-diabetes. Findings from the third National Health and Nutrition Examination Survey J Clin Endocrinol Metab. 2011; 96(9): 2898–2903.

St-Onge MP. Are normal-weight Americans over-fat? Obesity (Silver Spring). 2010; 18(11): 2067–2068.

St-Onge MP, Janssen I, Heymsfield SB. Metabolic syndrome in normal-weight Americans: new definition of the metabolically obese, normal-weight individual. Diabetes Care. 2004; 27(9): 2222–2228.

Stenholm S, Harris TB, Rantanen T, Visser M, Kritchevsky SB, Ferrucci L. Sarcopenic obesity: definition, etiology, and consequences. Curr Opin Clin Nutr Metab Care. 2008; 11(6): 693–700.

Stewart AE, Lord JH. Motor vehicle crash versus accident: a change in terminology is necessary. J Trauma Stress. 2002; 15(4): 333–335.

Suganami T, Ogawa Y. Role of chronic inflammation in adipose tissue in the pathophysiology of obesity. Nihon Rinsho. 2013; 71(2): 225–230.

Sundgot-Borgen J, Torstveit MK. Aspects of disordered eating continuum in elite high-intensity sports. Scand J Med Sci Sports. 2010; 20 Suppl 2: 112–121.

Szivak T, Hooper D, Dunn-Lewis C, et al. Adrenal cortical responses to high intensity, short rest, resistance exercise in men and women. J Strength Cond Res. 2013; 27(3): 748–760.

Tack CJ, Stienstra R, Joosten LA, Netea MG. Inflammation links excess fat to insulin resistance: the role of the interleukin-1 family. Immunol Rev. 2012; 249(1): 239–252.

Tailor A, Ogden J. Avoiding the term 'obesity': an experimental study of the impact of doctors' language on patients' beliefs. Patient Educ Couns. 2009; 76(2): 260–264.

Tanamas SK, Ng WL, Backholer K, Hodge A, Zimmet PZ, Peeters A. Quantifying the proportion of deaths due to body mass index- and waist circumference-defined obesity. Obesity (Silver Spring) 2016; 24(3): 735–742.

Templeman NM, Skovsø S, Page MM, Lim GE, Johnson JD. A causal role for hyperinsulinemia in obesity. J Endocrinol. 2017; 232(3): R173-R183.

Tomiyama AJ, Hunger JM, Nguyen-Cuu J, Wells C. Misclassification of cardiometabolic health when using body mass index categories in NHANES 2005–2012. Int J Obes (Lond). 2016; 40(5): 883–886.

Trappe S, Harber M, Creer A, et al. Single muscle fiber adaptations with marathon training. J Appl Physiol (1985). 2006; 101(3): 721–727.

Trayhurn P, Beattie JH. Physiological role of adipose tissue: white adipose tissue as an endocrine and secretory organ. Proc Nutr Soc. 2001; 60(3): 329–339.

Tucker AM, Vogel RA, Lincoln AE, et al. Prevalence of cardiovascular disease risk factors among National Football League players. JAMA. 2009; 301(20): 2111–2119.

Unger RH. Longevity, lipotoxicity and leptin: the adipocyte defense against feasting and famine. Biochimie. 2005; 87(1): 57–64.

University of Houston. Body Composition (http://www.uh.edu/fitness/PPTs/bodycomp.pdf).

van de Vyver M, Engelbrecht L, Smith C, Myburgh KH. Neutrophil and monocyte responses to downhill running: intracellular contents of MPO, IL-6, IL-10, pstat3, and SOCS3. Scand J Med Sci Sports. 2016; 26(6): 638–647.

Vatanparast H, Chilibeck PD, Cornish SM, et al. DXA-derived abdominal fat mass, waist circumference, and blood lipids in postmenopausal women. Obesity (Silver Spring). 2009; 17(8): 1635–1640.

Volek JS, Freidenreich DJ, Saenz C, et al. Metabolic characteristics of keto-adapted ultra-endurance runners. Metabolism. 2016; 65(3): 100–110.

Volek JS, Noakes T, Phinney SD. Rethinking fat as a fuel for endurance exercise. Eur J Sport Sci. 2015; 15(1): 13–20.

von Haehling S, Anker SD. Prevalence, incidence and clinical impact of cachexia: facts and numbers—update 2014. J Cachexia Sarcopenia Muscle. 2014; 5(4): 261–263.

Walsh NP, Gleeson M, Shephard RJ, et al. Position statement part one: immune function and exercise. Exerc Immunol Rev. 2011; 17: 6–63.

Weiss R, Bremer AA, Lustig RH. What is metabolic syndrome, and why are children getting it? Ann N Y Acad Sci. 2013; 1281: 123–140.

Yancy WS, Olsen MK, Guyton JR, Bakst RP, Westman EC. A low-carbohydrate, ketogenic diet versus a low-fat diet to treat obesity and hyperlipidemia: a randomized, controlled trial. Ann Intern Med. 2004; 140(10): 769–777.